PERFUMES, SPLASHES & COLOGNES

DISCOVERING AND CRAFTING
YOUR PERSONAL FRAGRANCES

NANCY M. BOOTH

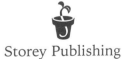
Storey Publishing

The mission of Storey Publishing is to serve our customers by publishing practical information that encourages personal independence in harmony with the environment.

Edited by Sonja Hakala and Deborah Balmuth
Copyedited by Ruth Sylvester
Cover design by Susan Bernier
Cover illustration by Laura Tedeschi
Text design and production by Susan Bernier (based on original design by
    Carol Jessop, Black Trout Design)
Production assistance by Erin Lincourt
Illustrations by Laura Tedeschi
Indexed by Susan Olason, Indexes & Knowledge Maps

The information in this book is true and complete to the best of our knowledge. All recommendations are made without guarantee on the part of the author or Storey Publishing. The author and publisher disclaim any liability in connection with the use of this information. For additional information please contact Storey Publishing, 210 MASS MoCA Way, North Adams, MA 01247.

Storey books are available for special premium and promotional uses and for customized editions. For further information, please call 1-800-793-9396.

Printed in the United States by Edwards Brothers, Inc.
20 19 18 17 16 15 14 13 12 11 10 9

Library of Congress Cataloging-in-Publication Data

Booth, Nancy M., 1947-
    Perfumes, splashes & colognes : discovering & crafting your personal
    fragrances / Nancy M. Booth.
            p.   cm.
    Includes bibliographical references and index.
    ISBN 978-0-88266-985-4 (pbk. : alk. paper)
    1. Perfumes. I. Title.
TP983.B66 1997
668'.54—dc21   97-26374
                                                                    CIP

TABLE OF CONTENTS

Introduction 1

Chapter 1:   The Essentials of Fragrance 10

Chapter 2:   The Ingredients of Fragrance 23

Chapter 3:   Building Your Fragrance Profile 47

Chapter 4:   How to Create Your Own Fragrances 65

Chapter 5:   Recipes for Perfumes, Colognes, and Sweet Waters . . .73

Chapter 6:   More Forms of Fragrance: Bath Salts,
             Incense, and More 111

Chapter 7:   Packaging Your Fragrances 129

Appendix A: Perfumes Listed by Fragrance Family 136

Appendix B: Perfumers and Their Perfumes .142

Appendix C: Fragrant Flowers and Their Scents 149

Source Guide 153

Related Reading Material 156

Glossary 157

Index 164

DEDICATION

To the family I love, husband Bill, son Christopher, daughter-in-law Maura, daughter Robin, and my sweet grandbabies, Victoria Leigh and Kyle Reed, and my mother-in-law, Jane Booth. You are the fabric of my life and treasured gifts from God. Thank you for surrounding me with the warmth of your love.

To Lynn, my childhood friend who has always been there to listen and share in all my joys and sorrows. Thanks for being the best friend this side of paradise. Love to your mother Mabs, my second Mom and stalwart supporter.

ACKNOWLEDGMENTS

My sincere thanks to Deborah Balmuth and Sonja Hakala, my editors, for their encouragement and enthusiasm, and to Storey Communications, for giving me the opportunity to write this book.

I could not have accomplished this task without the computer skills of my son Christopher and daughter-in-law Maura, daughter Robin, and friend Diane Nicholas.

Caswell-Massey's Jean Rettig-Carr was most generous with samples and information on America's oldest chemists and perfumers. Andrew D. Puckering, from Floris of London, also supplied me with facts about this purveyor of English flower perfumes.

I'd also like to thank Heather Maier, Chanel's counter manager at Macy's (Montgomery Mall, PA); Dolly Millard, Nordstrom's (King of Prussia, PA) fragrance consultant; and Janis Bader of Bloomingdale's (Willow Grove Mall, PA) for their generous sharing of time and information. They provided not only valuable knowledge but also samples of the newest perfumes. Dolly invited me to Nordstrom's special fragrance events. It was here that I met and spoke to Jean Kerléo, perfumer for Jean Patou.

I had the privilege of meeting Annette Green, president of the Fragrance Foundation in New York; the FF's library and Ms. Green's symposium at the Ritz Carlton provided invaluable information.

I'd also like to thank Bernard Zimmerman, Director of Application Resource for the Ungerer Co. in Lincoln Park, NJ. He has been a friend for nearly twenty years and his help with technical information on ingredients and the structure and composition of perfume deserves a special thank you.

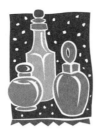

INTRODUCTION

When I was eight years old, I was given an F.A.O. Schwartz Christmas catalog with instructions to pick out a gift for myself. I selected a perfume kit for blending your own scents. When Christmas morning arrived and my miniature perfume laboratory lay waiting under the tree, I was sure I would be able to give Coco Chanel a run for her money! I spent many a happy hour concocting fragrant mixtures and giving them names like Midnight Magic, Moonbeams and Roses, and Clouds of Kisses. (Remember I was only eight.) I colored my creations pink, blue, lavender, and green, then added flowers from our gardens. (Yes, I was ahead of the times.) Eventually, I used dark red, fragrant roses from our gardens to color my mixtures and I pressed violets in order to adhere them to the outsides of my little bottles, as well as adding them to my perfumes.

As a teenager, I haunted perfume counters, eager to try new scents. I still remember with great fondness a scent called Majorca created by Revlon which came in a milkglass bottle with green accents. Later in my life, as a young mother with small children, I stopped at the local department store to practice with the newest make-up shades and fragrances. Sometimes, I was fragrantly overwhelming, causing my children to roll down the car windows. But I always felt my day was a success if I went home with a sample or two.

As my children grew and I decided to go back to work, I settled upon the idea of starting a fragrance business concentrating on scents and products to enhance the home. I truly believe that fragrance enhances your living space and your person.

Of all our senses, smell triggers the strongest memories. For example, the smell of cookies baking may trigger memories of a favorite grandmother, or the scent of lavender may remind you of your father. The scent of strawberry jam may take you back to leisurely Sunday morning breakfasts spent lolling over the newspaper while a combination of cotton candy and salty sea spray might remind you of a summer on the boardwalk. As we discuss fragrance in this book, keep in mind the smells which bring back pleasant thoughts for you and try to recreate them within your "scent-sual" environment.

THE HISTORY OF PERFUME

Perfume has an ancient and honorable lineage. As early as 4000 B.C., fragrant substances were burned in China, Arabia, and Egypt for sacred purposes, their smoke thought to carry messages to the deities. In the early Egyptian civilization, certain scents were considered more precious than gold and some of their unguent jars, opened after thousands of years, still retained their fragrance. The use of these incenses spread among the ancient Greek and Roman civilizations. Fragrance gradually became valued for personal use and people began to wear fragrance to evoke behavioral responses or to enhance their status.

The word perfume is from the Latin phrase "per fumum," meaning "through smoke."

Burning Fragrance

Incense is made of a combination of resins, fragrant woods, and gums in solid or powdered forms. In ancient Egypt, people burned *kyphi* in their temples and homes. This sacred perfume was an incense paste made of a wine and raisin base with the addition of aromatic herbs and resins.

After the fall of Roman civilization in 476 A.D., the use of personal fragrance in Europe declined until the Renaissance. As it was for arts and letters, the Renaissance was a brilliant period for fragrance development. The use of essential oils expanded to include spices such as cloves, nutmeg, and mace. Early perfumers created aromatic waters from scents such as orange and rose and began to use animal fixatives such as ambergris, civet, and musk.

In 1370, the first alcohol-based perfume was created for Queen Elizabeth of Hungary. Elizabeth, well known for her great beauty, was 72 when a Polish king of twenty-five asked for her hand in marriage. The recipe for Hungary water, said to be responsible for preserving Elizabeth's great beauty, is still manufactured today. Directions to make this historical fragrance are included in chapter 5.

The French trace their notable passion for perfume back to 1533 and the arrival of Catherine de Médici from Italy to marry their king, Henry II. Catherine was responsible for setting up the first perfume laboratory at Grasse, near the Mediterranean coast. Now, four centuries later, this region of the world is still famous as an international center of fragrance and flower production.

By the sixteenth century, Grasse, France, was also a center for the leather tanning industry. Leather gloves from Grasse were perfumed with amber, spices, jasmine, frangipani, and musk so that women and men could hold them to their noses while walking in streets where sewage ran in the gutter. When the leather business declined during the eighteenth century, the makers of perfumed gloves switched to manufacturing just perfumes, creating scented pomades from orange flowers gathered from trees planted for that purpose.

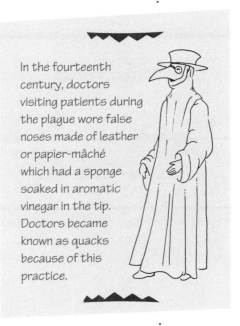

In the fourteenth century, doctors visiting patients during the plague wore false noses made of leather or papier-mâché which had a sponge soaked in aromatic vinegar in the tip. Doctors became known as quacks because of this practice.

Louis XIV (1638–1715) of France became known as the Perfume King (Le Roi Parfum) as well as the Sun King (Le Roi Soleil). He required members of his court to wear a different perfume every day, which he selected. At that time, perfume was reserved for the nobility and was often kept in beautiful, one-of-a-kind bottles.

Modern perfumery began in 1806 with the marketing of Eau de Cologne by Jean Maria Farina. His formula, which originated in Cologne, Germany, was patented in 1818 and consisted of an alcohol-water base scented with an oil composed of neroli, bergamot, rosemary, and lemon. This alcohol-based formula evaporated quickly, leaving a pleasantly clean citrus scent behind. Roger et Gallet, which took over the Farina perfume house, still produces the original Eau de Cologne today.

There was an American version of Eau de Cologne called Florida Water trademarked in New York by Murray and Lanman in 1808. True to its name, it uses a citrus (hesperidium) base with bergamot, lavender, and clove. There's a Florida Water recipe on page 79.

A Scent(sual) History

Before 1925, the coveted perfumes of France were sold exclusively in the major salons of Paris, but by 1930 the distribution of French fragrance extended to the United States. At that time American fashion designers began to develop their own lines of fine perfumes just as today's ready-to-wear designers do. The days of one-of-a-kind, custom perfumes created for the rich are long gone. Today there's a fragrance for everyone, for every feeling, mood, activity and lifestyle.

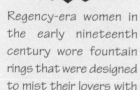

Regency-era women in the early nineteenth century wore fountain rings that were designed to mist their lovers with perfume as they bent to kiss their lady's hand.

While most people don't know how perfume is made, they do know what pleases their nose. This is a short history of some of the world's most famous perfumes and their creators. There are more perfumers listed in the appendix on page 142.

Arpège

Jeanne Lanvin launched Arpège in 1925. This famous perfume is a combination of bergamot, neroli, rose, jasmine, ylang ylang, sandalwood, patchouli, and vanilla, all enhanced by aldehydes. Arpège is one of the top ten fragrances in the world.

Chanel No. 5

Chemist Ernest Beaux created Chanel No. 5 for Paris fashion designer Gabrielle (Coco) Chanel in May 1921. The brilliant sparkle of this aldehydic fragrance added a new dimension to perfumery with its unique composition, and Chanel No. 5 remains one of the best selling perfumes in the world. Chanel named her signature scent No. 5 because an astrologer told Coco that five was her lucky number. Its popularity soared when Marilyn Monroe remarked "the only thing she wore to bed was a little Chanel No. 5."

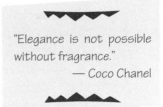

"Elegance is not possible without fragrance."
— Coco Chanel

Chypre

François Coty was quite an innovator in the world of perfumes. In 1905, he produced L'Origan (oregano) which started a trend towards spicy florals. But in 1917, when Coty launched a perfume called Chypre, he launched a whole new family of scent. Oakmoss, patchouli, labdanum, bergamot, calamus, clary sage, sandalwood, and vetiver are typical components in a chypre blend.

Eau Neuve

This perfume, created by Jean-François Lubin in 1798, was originally named Pauline in honor of Napoleon Bonaparte's sister, the Princess Pauline Borghese. Lubin operated a boutique in Paris, Aux Armes de France, which was famous for its delicious lotions, perfumed milk powders, smelling salts, and lovely toilet articles. Composed of lavender, civet, and citronella, Pauline's time honored formula was used to create Eau Neuve in 1968.

Femme

During the 1930s, Marcel Rochas was Hollywood's favorite designer. Carole Lombard, Marlene Dietrich, and Jean Harlow were just a few of the stars who flocked to his salon. Edmond Roudnitska, who became a very famous nose in the perfume industry, created Femme for Rochas in 1944. Femme contains peach and plum blended with grasses, jasmine, rose, amber, patchouli, and musk. This fragrance dominated the 1950s and helped fuel the popularity of the chypre perfumes pioneered by François Coty.

Joy

Jean Patou earned his place in the perfume hall of fame with the creation of the incredibly expensive and still revered perfume Joy. Large quantities of jasmine and Bulgarian rose form the body of this incomparable fragrance. It has been referred to as "the costliest perfume in the world" since its introduction in 1929.

Quality control is difficult in the world of perfume because the international gardens which produce the flowers and essences for use in fragrance experience differing growing conditions from year to year. Great perfumers such as Jean Kerléo of the House of Patou regularly visit the rose plantations of Egypt, France, Turkey, and Bulgaria to choose flowers which will exactly replicate the fragrance of perfumes such as Joy.

FAMOUS BOTTLES

Perfumes are often prized as much for their unusual containers, called flacons, as for the scents inside. Of all perfume bottle designers, René Lalique is probably the most famous. He designed the cooing doves on the stopper of L'Air du Temps, which was launched by Nina Ricci in 1948. The curve of Lalique's bottle for Femme, created by perfumer Edmond Roudnitska in 1944, is inspired by the curve of Mae West's hips.

In 1906, Lalique was approached by François Coty to design flacons for the perfumer's creations. This long creative collaboration, which produced 16 flacons in all, started with a container for L'Effleurt which features a genie rising from swirling vapors and veils that curl up from honeysuckle petals.

Salvador Dali, the best known of the surrealist painters, hopped into the perfume business with his usual aplomb and sense of humor. In 1983, he introduced his own fragrance called, appropriately enough, Salvador Dali. The perfume, a floral aldehyde blend, is wonderful but the bottle is a knockout. The base of Dali's flacon is a very full set of smiling lips and the stopper is a somewhat aquiline nose. The design was taken from Dali's painting L'Aphrodite de Cnide.

L'Air du Temps

Nina Ricci, a fashion designer with a flair for romantic clothes, opened her perfume business in 1945. Under her son Robert's direction, L'air du Temps was created in 1948 and it's still one of the top five perfumes in the world. The bottle's beautiful design, by René Lalique, features two doves with their wings lifted. Some of L'Air du Temps' ingredients include jasmine, carnation, sandalwood, gardenia, irisantheme, carnation, rose, ylang ylang, musk, and ambergris, which together create a floral blend with spicy undertones.

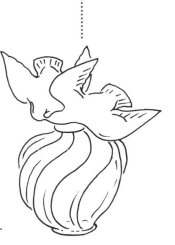

Quelques Fleurs

The perfumery opened in 1775 by Jean-François Houbigant is still creating fabulous fragrances today. In 1912 Houbigant's perfumer, Monsieur Bienaimé, created Quelques Fleurs (a few flowers) suffused with an amber bouquet. It was reintroduced in 1985 under the name Quelques Fleurs L'Original. It is a landmark perfume, the first true multifloral fragrance. It has notes of jasmine, rose, violet, and lilac.

During the 19th century, most perfumes were single flower types, such as rose, violet, or lavender, fixed with natural civet, musk, and ambergris. Houbigant's Quelques Fleurs changed this practice by including a blend of more than one scent.

> Chantilly is an old and well-loved amber from Houbigant. It was named for a French town famous for horseracing. The perfume is as feminine as the French lace of the same name.

Shalimar

Pierre-François Guerlain established his family's perfume business in 1828. After his death in 1864, Guerlain's sons continued the family tradition and it was under their leadership, in 1889, that the perfumery produced its first well-known scent, Jicky. However, this sparkling scent's renown was eclipsed by the famous Shalimar in 1925 when Jacques Guerlain poured a sample of synthetic vanilla into a bottle of Jicky. The resulting fragrance was incredible. Over seventy years have passed since

Shalimar's introduction and it still accounts for seventeen percent of Guerlain's sales.

Vent Vert

When it was introduced in 1947, fashion designer Pierre Balmain described Vent Vert as "an exhilarating fragrance, evoca-
tive of nature in spring." Vent Vert means "green breeze" in
French and this perfume was the first in a line of sharp, green
fragrances with the scent of leaves, sap, and dewy spring flowers. One of the great female perfumers, Germaine Cellier, created Vent Vert.

Youth Dew

Estée Lauder's innovations transformed the world of American
perfumery. In 1953, she introduced Youth Dew essence in the
form of bath oil and it revolutionized the way American women
looked at perfume. Youth Dew is an exotic combination of bergamot, geranium, and chamomile, along with the rich floral
scents of rose, jasmine, muguet, and ylang ylang blended
against a background of sandalwood, vetiver, and patchouli.

Lauder went on to create many scents such as Private Collection. In 1996, Lauder's perfume Pleasures won the American
Star of the Year award at the Fragrance Foundation FIFI award
ceremony in New York City.

PERFUMERY'S VERSION OF AMBER

No, perfumes do not include a powdered form of the familiar, honey-colored gem-
stone prized as a jewel. To perfumers, amber has three meanings. It can be used to
refer to ambergris, a substance which originates in the sperm whale and is used as
a fixative in perfume. Amber also describes the aroma of labdanum, a fragrant oleoresin derived from rockroses. And it is also used to describe commercial perfumes
which have a dramatic, warm, and powdery scent.

THE POWER OF SCENT IN EVERYDAY LIFE

Since I am in the fragrance business, scent plays an important part in my life, as I'm certain it does in yours. Compare your scent-sual day to mine.

As I shower, I notice the scent of my shampoo and shower gel. Fresh peppermint toothpaste is a wake-up call and I apply a spritz of fragrance with matching dusting powder while I dress.

Before I hop in my car, I make a detour to the garden to see what flowers or herbs opened that morning. As the spring blossoms fade, lilacs and peonies bloom. June's arrival brings my beloved roses in all their glory. (For information about fragrant flowers and their sources, see the appendix on page 149.)

> "Perfume is like love, you can never get enough of it."
> —Estée Lauder

When I arrive at Gingham 'n' Spice, Ltd., I am positively surrounded by aromas. Our checks and stationery become imbued with a medley of fragrances. The bank always knows who's making a deposit when my checks arrive.

One of the things I love best about my husband Bill is that he always smells wonderful! When we leave for work, he smells crisp and fresh. But he sometimes carries another cologne in his briefcase so he may return smelling of vanilla, sandalwood, and spice. He slips into bed wearing Realm for Men, hopeful the pheromones will "bring the honeybee to the honey."

When I return home in the evening, I light scented candles. When I change the sheets, scented dusting powder is sprinkled on the mattress and there are lavender sachets in the linen closet. As I get ready for bed, the last thing I do is hydrate my skin with rosewater after removing my makeup. Then it's a light spray of scent on my nightie and I'm at the end of another day.

As you go through your day, notice how many products you use because you like their scent. Do you stoop down to smell the flowers in the grocery store or breathe in deep when you approach a bakery? Notice how you react to certain smells. How do they make you feel? Once you begin to notice fragrance, you'll begin to realize how important it is to your life.

CHAPTER 1

THE ESSENTIALS OF FRAGRANCE

Fragrances are divided into families or categories of similar types of aromas. As you set out to choose a fragrance, start by listing scents you have worn and enjoyed or aromas which please your nose. Then find out which fragrance family these scents belong to. Usually, you will find a similarity in your choices. If your selections fall into different categories, choose your absolute favorite and explore that fragrance family or try several from each family that you like.

FRAGRANCE FAMILIES FOR WOMEN

The floral family is by far the largest scent category and the most popular. Others include Fruity, Green, Spicy, Floriental, Oriental, Citrus, Modern, Chypre and Ozone-Oceanic.

Floral

Examples of scents in this category include rose, lily of the valley, carnation, narcissus, gardenia, tuberose, and violet. Floral perfumes are usually combinations of several different scents. Some of the more famous floral perfumes include Jardins de Bagatelle (Guerlain), Joy (Patou), L'Air du Temps (Nina Ricci), and Chanel No. 22 (Chanel).

There is a subcategory of perfumes in the floral fragrance family in which the predominant scent is of one particular flower.

SINGLE FLORAL PERFUMES

Flower	Perfume
Rose	Tea Rose (Perfumer's Workshop)
Lily of the Valley	Diorissimo (Dior)
Carnation	Bellodgia (Caron)
Narcissus	Narcisse Noir (Caron)
Gardenia	Gardenia Passion (Annick Goutal)
Tuberose	Chloe (Lagerfeld)
Violet	Vera Violetta (Roger & Gallet)

Fruity

The fruity family of scents includes mandarin, neroli, nectarine, papaya, bergamot, apple, apricot, melon, passion fruit, and pineapple. Fruity scents have a clean, fresh citrus-like quality and a smooth, mellow peach-like warmth. Some well-known fruity perfumes include Lauren (Ralph Lauren) which smells of pineapple, Il Bacio (Borghese) with its mixture of peach, plum, melon, pear, and passion fruit, and Laura Ashley No. 1 (Laura Ashley) which smells of peach and bergamot.

Green

Love the smell of freshly cut grass and new green leaves? This family includes fragrances such as pine, juniper, hyacinth, galbanum, lavender, and rosemary. Some excellent examples of perfumes in the green family include Vent Vert (Balmain), Cabotine (Grès), Chanel No. 19 (Chanel), and Aliage (Lauder).

Spicy

This family includes the scents of cinnamon, cloves, ginger, and cardamom plus flowers such as carnations and lavender which have spicy notes in them. Spicy perfumes include Nahema (Guerlain), KL (Lagerfeld), Dioressence (Dior), and Cinnabar (Lauder).

Floriental

Strictly speaking, floriental is not a fragrance family. But this subcategory is important enough to warrant mention. It includes scents that are lighter than those found in the oriental family, appropriate for daytime as well as evening wear. Spices, balsams, and resins combine with exotic floral essences to produce floriental blends. Perfumes in this subcategory include Chanel's Allure, Trésor by Lancôme, Venezia from Laura Biagiotti, Samsara from Guerlain, and Arden's Fifth Avenue. St. John eau de parfum, from a designer of the same name, is a delicious floriental with top notes of freesia, tangerine, osmanthus, and orange flower with a heart of miel (honey), moonflower, gardenia, jasmine, and honeysuckle resting on a base of apricot, sandalwood, amber, and musk.

Oriental

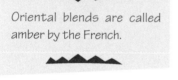

Oriental blends are called amber by the French.

This is the heaviest fragrance group and is most appropriate for evening wear. It includes woods, resins, musk, amber, and vanilla. Some of the finest oriental perfumes include Shalimar (Guerlain), Bal à Versailles (Desprez), Opium (St. Laurent), and Obsession (Calvin Klein).

Citrus

These light, fresh scents include the aroma of lemons, limes, grapefruit, mandarin, and bergamot. Some classic citrus perfumes include Eau d'Hadrien (Annick Goutal), Eau de Patou, and Eau de Cologne Impériale still sold by Guerlain in the original bottle with an imperial bee motif done in gold.

Modern

These blends contain aldehydes, which are pure aroma chemicals. They add sparkle and a fragrance that intensifies as it is warmed on the skin. The aldehydes also amplify the other scents in a perfume. The first aldehydic fragrance was Chanel

No. 5 and other examples of perfumes in the modern family include Arpège (Lanvin), White Linen (Lauder), and Madame Rochas (Rochas).

Because aldehydes enhance the scent of perfumes, their use in perfumery has expanded since their introduction in 1921. Nowadays, almost all perfumes contain aldehydes.

Chypre

François Coty inspired this family of scents when he introduced a perfume by this name in 1917. Chypre was named for the Mediterranean Island of Cypress and has a woodsy-mossy bouquet characterized by notes of lavender, oakmoss, patchouli, clary sage, and resins. Wonderful examples of chypre perfumes are Ysatis (Givenchy), Miss Dior (Dior), Cabochard (Grès), and Jolie Madame (Balmain).

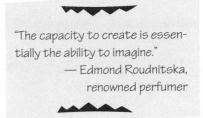

"The capacity to create is essentially the ability to imagine."
— Edmond Roudnitska, renowned perfumer

Ozone-Oceanic

This is the newest family of scent and it is based wholly on synthetic materials that remind people of sea spray, fresh mountain air, and the fragrance of just-washed linen. Good examples of perfumes in this family include Dune (Dior), L'Eau d'Issey (Issey Miyake), Sunflowers (Arden), and Acqua di Giō (Armani).

FRAGRANCE FAMILIES FOR MEN

Tests conducted on men at the Smell and Taste Treatment and Research Foundation are interesting. The most arousing scents were a combination of pumpkin pie and lavender followed by doughnuts and licorice. Green apple was considered relaxing while the most popular aroma in the single scent category was orange.

While there are no doughnut-scented fragrances for men, there are several wonderful scents to choose from. Men's fragrances fall into six different families or classifications. Some of them are similar to the fragrance families for women and some are unique for men.

Citrus

The citrus family is often described as fresh and brisk. Scents in the citrus family are made from the oils of lemons, limes, oranges, and the fruit of the bergamot tree. Examples of citrus fragrances for men include Eau Sauvage (Dior), Eternity (Calvin Klein), Eau de Cologne Impériale (Guerlain), and Polo Sport (Lauren).

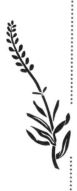

Spicy

This highly popular scent family for men incorporates nutmeg, cinnamon, cloves, pepper, bay oil from the West Indies, Mediterranean basil, and olibanum. Examples of fragrance in the spicy family for men include JHL (Lauder/Aramis), Egoïste (Chanel), Jaguar (Frey), and Old Spice (Shulton). Old Spice was introduced in 1937 and is still a favorite.

Leather

This fragrance family is based on a smoky, pungent, somewhat sweet scent that is very potent. Leather scents are created from cade oil, which comes from juniper trees, and birch tar, a resin extracted from birch trees growing in Finland. Examples of the leather family of fragrances for men include English Leather (Mem Co.), Pour Lui (Oscar de la Renta), Bel Ami (Hermès), and Lanvin for Men (Lanvin).

Lavender

This is one of the oldest scents in the fragrance world, made from oils extracted from the lavender and lavandin plants grown in France as well as spike lavender grown in Spain. Examples of fragrances in the lavender fragrance family for men include Old English Lavender (Yardley), Pour un Homme (Caron), Pino Silvestre (Vidal), and Le Male (Jean Paul Gaultier).

Fougère

In addition to anchoring a fragrance family of its own, lavender is a key accord in fougère fragrances. Fougère, pronounced fooz-hare, is French for "fern," which of course has no scent. In fragrance terminology, however, the fougère family is defined as a blend of oak moss, lavender, and the new-mown-hay smell of coumarin. Geranium oil appears in these blends too. Examples of the fougère fragrance family include Drakkar Noir (Laroche), Equipage (Hermès), Tuscany (Aramis/ Lauder), and Insatiable (Pierre Cardin).

Woody

The classic scents in this family are based on vetiver, cedar, rosewood, and sandalwood. Examples include XS (Paco Rabanne), Aramis (Aramis), Boucheron (Boucheron), and Safari (Lauren). While it is considered a member of the woody fragrance family, Grey Flannel (Geoffrey Beene), is dominated by the scent of violets. Kenzo Pour Homme (Kenzo) straddles a line in the fragrance families because it is considered an oceanic woody fragrance with clean, crisp accords of cedar, sandalwood, vetiver, musk, myrtle, and rare blue iris.

A WORD ABOUT SHARED SCENTS

Unisex fragrances, which are usually from the chypre family, are nothing new, yet perfumers are introducing new versions of fragrance for both genders all the time. The London perfumer Creed, established in 1760, continues its centuries-old tradition with such unisex eau de toilettes as Baie de Genievrie, a berry and juniper blend, and Orange Spice. The label for Royal Delight, a favorite of Queen Victoria, quietly illustrates the point about unisex fragrances. It depicts a man and woman together on horseback. In 1966, Eau Sauvage started the unisex toilet water rage and cK one was a rousing success upon its introduction in 1995 by Calvin Klein.

Unisex fragrances sometimes come in complementary versions such as St Laurent's Opium and Opium for Men. Tommy Hilfiger's tommy has its counterpart in tommy girl and Hermès has a dynamic duo in Calèche for her and Bel Ami for him.

Did you know that babies have an inborn ability to recognize their mother's scents? Jacadi, a French company, has a collection based on the theory that sharing fragrance stimulates mother/child closeness. Eau des Petites (0–2 years) contains no alcohol and has a very light scent. Eau des Grands (2–10) 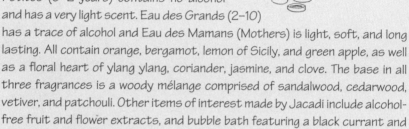 has a trace of alcohol and Eau des Mamans (Mothers) is light, soft, and long lasting. All contain orange, bergamot, lemon of Sicily, and green apple, as well as a floral heart of ylang ylang, coriander, jasmine, and clove. The base in all three fragrances is a woody mélange comprised of sandalwood, cedarwood, vetiver, and patchouli. Other items of interest made by Jacadi include alcohol-free fruit and flower extracts, and bubble bath featuring a black currant and apricot accord.

Other perfumes for the youngest scent-wearers include Annick Goutal's Eau de Bonpoint, a lovely creation of orange blossom and neroli softened by rosewood and vanilla, Givenchy's Pitsenbon and Guerlain's Petit Guerlain.

FRAGRANCE AND ESSENTIAL OILS

The building blocks of all fragrance are the essential oils extracted from flowers, grasses, seeds, leaves, roots, barks, fruits, mosses, and resins. In recent years, these pure plant distillates have themselves become popular, appearing on the shelves of health food and other specialty stores from coast to coast. They are very concentrated and because their production demands large quantities of raw material, they can be quite expensive.

In some cases, a flower or fruit may not give up its fragrance in an essential oil. For example, the scent of lily of the valley or pears is impossible to distill in an essential oil. Over the years, the perfume industry has created synthetics to duplicate these scents while expanding the fragrance frontier to include compounds that smell like salty sea air. Natural and synthetic fragrant sources complement each other — the new aromatics contribute special and unusual notes to a perfume while essential oils round out, fix, and soften a compound — and both are indispensable to modern perfumery.

Essential oils are extracted in a variety of ways including distillation, expression, solvent extraction, and enfleurage. Different plants, because of their individual properties, call for different extraction methods. For example, the oils in citrus materials such as oranges, limes, and bergamot are usually expressed (forced out by pressure) because the fragrant part of the plant is the peel. The essence of lavender, on the other hand, is captured by distillation.

Often the creation and manufacture of a perfume calls for fragrant materials that are even more concentrated than essential oils. Concretes are a semi-solid, waxy substance extracted from essential oils by volatile solvents. Their odor is closest to the original plant material. Concretes can be further concentrated, usually by alcohol extraction, to produce absolutes, the most concentrated form of perfumery material.

The essential oils of many plants are derived through distillation. For example, if you wanted to extract oil from chamomile, you would submerge the flowers in boiling water, then capture and cool the resulting steam. Once the steam condenses back to water, the oil separates from it, resting on the surface to await collection.

In perfumery, this distillation process serves two functions. It not only separates essential oils from plant material, it concentrates and purifies the result. By the way, the water left behind with the plant material is often sold as sweet water.

Another common method of extracting essential oils is enfleurage. This process originated in ancient Egypt and uses cold purified fats to extract a flower's oils. The fatty result of enfleurage is called pomade. An alcohol solvent is applied to the pomade to extract the essential oil. This method is very costly but it produces the finest jasmine, rose, and violet oils.

COMPOSING A PERFUME

Traditionally, perfume is a blend of natural, essential oils extracted from spices, herbs, flowers, grasses, leaves, and woods to which scent-prolonging fixatives are added. Modern perfumes are a concentrated essence of fragrant materials, including various synthetic ingredients, diluted in the smallest possible amount of high-grade alcohol. The more deluxe fragrances have a higher ratio of natural materials to synthetic ingredients. In addition to the correct blend of scented materials, a fine fragrance must be properly filtered and matured. It must also be safe to use on the skin.

There are approximately 3,000 raw ingredients available to choose from when perfumers compose a fragrance. When they talk about this process, perfumers use the terms top, middle, and base notes to describe the different elements which make up a perfume's overall essence.

In the nineteenth century, French perfumer Septimus Piésse implemented a classification system for perfume which corresponds to the musical scale. He described perfumes as thematic with each note carrying a common thread. In fact, Piésse compared octaves of odor to those in musical composition. In Piésse's classification system, which is still used today, each odor is assigned a different musical note on a scale. If a perfume is formulated correctly, the final symphony of scent, from its original application to the skin through drydown, will contain all the right chords.

In 1923, a man named W. A. Poucher added to the work of Piésse when he published a classification method based on a fragrant ingredient's evaporation rate. Based on an overall scale of 1 to 100, Poucher assigned top notes to the numbers 1 through 15 because they evaporate

OF NOTES, THREADS, AND OCTAVES

A fragrance composition contains individual notes or essences. The term "notes" can refer to a single ingredient such as jasmine, frankincense, or lemon but may also refer to a perfume's phase or a fragrant blend of ingredients that combine to give a perfume its top, middle, or base notes.

The term "common thread" describes a perfume's ability to flow from one phase to another in a cohesive rather than a discordant fashion.

And a perfume's "octave" refers to the height of a particular odor or ingredient as it makes its presence known during the drydown process.

quickly. For example, mandarin is a 2, coriander is a 3, and nutmeg an 11. Middle notes are rated from 16 to 69 and include ingredients such as marjoram (18), clovebud (22), and jonquil absolute and ylang-ylang (both of which are 24). Rose, tuberose, and jasmine absolute are all rated 43.

Base note fragrances, which last the longest, are rated from 70 to 100 and include galbanum and opopanax resins at 90, angelica at 94, and many valuable fixatives rated at 100. Those with the highest rating, meaning they last the longest and evaporate the slowest, include frankincense, benzoin, patchouli, sandalwood, oakmoss, tonka bean, and vetiver. Poucher's classification system was updated in 1991 and is still used by perfumers as a guideline when composing a fragrance.

Historically, when a perfumer, who is called the "Nose" in the industry, set out to create a new fragrance, he or she began work at a structure called an organ. It consisted of a series of curved, stepped shelves, similar in shape to a church organ, lined with essential oils arranged by scent categories such as citrus or spice. A perfumer would also have a large number of specialty bases, which are ready-made accords of synthetic and natural oils.

Today few perfumers work at an organ. Instead, perfumes are created in the laboratory. The modern perfumer, who is still referred to in the industry as a Nose, begins with a product profile from a client. This profile outlines the client's conception of a fragrance, its price parameters plus ideas for the style, packaging, and type of customer to be targeted. With all the competition in the perfume industry, it is crucial that the perfume, packaging, and name all complement each other.

Top Notes

Top notes (notes de tête) are the lightest and most fleeting part of a perfume, providing the initial fragrance impression. Their initial appearance lasts but a few minutes but then they blend with the middle notes as that phase of the perfume begins. This is where the term "accord" comes from. It is a harmonious blending of the various notes. Just as there are more ingredients in the floral fragrance family, there are more fragrance sources in the top note classification than either the middle or base note groups.

Floral
geranium • chamomile
gardenia • tagetes (marigold)

Fruity
peach • pear • plum
apricot • raspberry • melon
black currant bud

Green
galbanum • hyacinth
lavender • rosemary • mint
basil • clary sage

Spices
**(sometimes appear
as top notes)**
cinnamon • cardamom
clove • coriander • pepper

Citrus
lemon • bergamot
petitgrain • lime • pineapple
neroli • mandarin
tangerine

Middle Notes

Middle notes (notes de cœur), define the character of a perfume, help classify its fragrance family, and can modify its base notes. It takes approximately ten minutes for middle notes, also called heart notes, to develop on the skin and they can last for hours, harmonizing with the supporting base notes. Middle notes tend to be rich in florals.

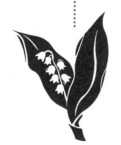

carnation • cyclamen • daffodil • frangipani
freesia • geranium • heliotrope • honey • honeysuckle
iris • jasmine • jonquil • lilac • lily of the valley
magnolia • mimosa • narcissus • orange blossom
orchid • peony • rose • stephanotis • sweet pea
tuberose • violet • water lily • white lily • ylang ylang

Base Notes

Base notes (notes de fond) carry the top and middle notes, giving a perfume its depth. Base notes are often referred to as fixatives because they prolong the evaporation rate, also called drydown, and the life of a fragrance on the skin.

ambergris • balsam • benzoin
castoreum • cedarwood • civet • coumarin
frankincense • labdanum • musk • myrrh
oakmoss • patchouli • resins
sandalwood • styrax • tonka bean
vanillin • vetiver

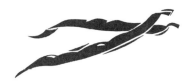

DRYDOWN PERIOD

Drydown occurs when the final phase of a fragrance develops on the skin. This usually takes a half an hour if the person wearing the perfume has dry skin and fifteen minutes if the skin is oily. Perfumers evaluate the tenacity of a fragrance during this stage.

THE DIFFERENCE BETWEEN FLOWERS AND THEIR SCENTS

From the moment a flower is picked or its petals gathered, its scent begins to change. But until recently, the type and rate of these changes could not be accurately tracked. Using a process called headspace analysis or living flower technology, chemists can now analyze the true scent of a living flower. International Flavor and Fragrance's Dr. Mookherjee discovered this technology in 1977 and described it as "touching the feet of God."

A domed bottle with a Tenax trap on one sidearm covers a living flower. Air is forced over the flower, and odor molecules are collected in the Tenax for analysis on a chromatograph. This analysis lets a chemist see how a living flower's scent differs from its extracted essential oil.

Perfumes designed with living flower technology include Floret (Antonia Bellanca), Calyx (Prescriptives), Evelyn (Crabtree & Evelyn), Parfum d'Été (Kenzo), Realm for Women (Erox Corp.), and Pleasures (Lauder).

In 1996, the IFF announced a further development in technology called Solid-Phase Micro Extraction. Although not originally developed by IFF, the foundation's Dr. Mookherjee adapted this process. It uses a fiber needle placed near a blossom or fruit to collect fragrance molecules. While a low-odor flower may have to be partially enclosed in a glass vessel, the fragrance of most flowers is collected while the plant is in the open. Once the odor chemicals are collected, a process which takes approximately two hours, the needle is injected into a spectrometer and the results analyzed.

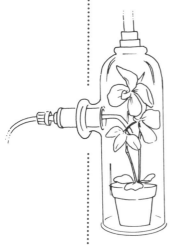

This new technology allows a flower's fragrance to be analyzed at different stages of its development. For example, when gardenias first open, they emit a fresh, green odor. Later, when all the petals are open, the flowers smell different, and after 24 hours, gardenia flowers have a much heavier, narcotic scent. Because of this technology, perfumers can now create variations of the same flower's scent.

Now that you have a little background on fragrance, let's move on to the wonderful ingredients that make up perfumes, colognes, and sweet waters so that you can make your own scents.

CHAPTER 2

THE INGREDIENTS OF FRAGRANCE

Commercial perfumes may contain as many as 300 ingredients such as essential oils, resins, and fixatives. While I didn't include every ingredient known to perfumery in this list, I did include information about perfumes that contain these ingredients so that you can more easily locate perfumes that include some of your favorite scents. I've also included, where appropriate, scents that complement each other when combined. This information will come in handy when you make your own fragrances.

ALLSPICE

In nature: This familiar baking spice is a combination of cloves, cinnamon, pepper, and juniper berries.

In perfume: Allspice lends a spicy note to several men's and women's fragrances. It's used as a top note in Lauder's Spellbound.

AMBER

In nature: Amber is often used by perfumers as a shortened form of the word ambergris, a material thought to be formed in the intestines of the sperm whale but found floating on the shores of the tropics. Amber is also used to describe the aroma of labdanum, a dark oleoresin derived from rockroses. The word amber is also used to identify the dramatic, warm, and powdery perfumes in the Oriental fragrance family.

In perfume: Since the sperm whale is an endangered species, only synthetic ambergris is used as a fixative in the perfume industry today.

ANGELICA

In nature: This essential oil is distilled from the roots and fruit of the Eurasian angelica plant.

In perfume: Angelica has a musky, benzoin odor and is sometimes used as a fixative, especially in chypre blends.

ANISE

In nature: The essential oil is distilled from the seed of this herbal relative of the carrot.

In perfume: Anise is usually used as a top note and it appears in Champagne by Yves St. Laurent.

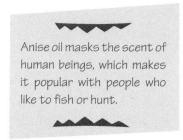

Anise oil masks the scent of human beings, which makes it popular with people who like to fish or hunt.

APPLE

In nature: Today, the scent of apples is obtained through synthesis or by distillation of their juice. Apple was a common scent in early perfumes developed in Arabia.

In perfume: Granny Smith apples were used by Perry Ellis in the creation of America for Women. Apple is also a top note in Escape by Calvin Klein.

APRICOT

In nature: The scent of apricots has never been successfully drawn from the fruit itself.

In perfume: Apricot scent is created synthetically for modern perfume and is often used to create fruity notes. It appears as a top note in Trésor by Lancôme.

APRICOT KERNEL OIL

In nature: While the scent of the fruit of an apricot has not been successfully drawn from the fruit, its seeds produce a golden oil with the lovely scent of apricots.

In perfume: While the kernel oil is not strong enough to be used as a fragrance material in perfume, it is an excellent choice as a carrier oil in fragrance crafting. Apricot kernel oil is also a good base oil for massage or to nourish dry, sensitive skin.

AZALEA

In nature: The vibrantly-colored azalea, familiar to so many gardeners, is not known for its fragrance. There are fragrant azaleas, however, but they are more scarce and do not give up their fragrance.

In perfume: Azalea fragrance is made synthetically for use in perfume.

BALSAM OF PERU

In nature: Balsam of Peru is extracted from the resinous material of trees now grown in El Salvador.

In perfume: There are several kinds of balsam. All have a vanilla-woody aroma, and are used as fixatives in perfume. V'E Versace perfume has balsamic base notes and Drakkar Noir by Laroche has a balsam base.

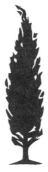

BASIL

In nature: As many gardeners know, there are several varieties of basil. The most common varieties cultivated for perfumery include the clove-scented *Ocimum sanctum* and the musky scented *Ocimum basilicum.*

In perfume: This sharp and spicy essential oil is used primarily as a middle note in perfume and resembles the fragrant flower mignonette. Guerlain's Jicky is a prime example of a perfume with a basil middle note.

BAY LEAF OIL

In nature: This warm, pungent, and spicy oil is distilled from the leaves of the European bay laurel.

In perfume: Bay leaf oil is frequently used in masculine scents and also as a base note in Galanos perfume for women or in Royall Bay Rhum for men.

BAYBERRY

In nature: Early European settlers in New England discovered the fragrant evergreen *Myrica cerifera* growing along Cape Cod Bay, but it also grows in the Bahamas, Bermuda, and the West Indies. When boiled, the berries and leaves yield a wax that is used in candlemaking.

In perfume: Synthetic bayberry is used in perfumery today.

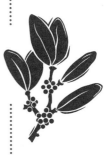

BENZOIN

In nature: Benzoin is a balsamic resin extracted from a tree known as the gum benjamin.

In perfume: Benzoin is used as a fixative and preservative. It is an important base note in Guerlain's Nahema.

BERGAMOT

In nature: This fresh, citrus-scented oil is expressed from an inedible fruit grown almost exclusively in Calabria, Italy.

In perfume: Essential to eau de colognes and a fine fixative, bergamot is found in the top notes of 34 percent of women's perfumes and 50 percent of men's fragrances. One example is Eau de Givenchy where it is the foremost top note in the composition. Bergamot oil is one of the oldest perfume ingredients.

BITTER ALMOND OIL

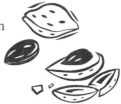

In nature: This essential oil is derived from the bitter almond tree.

In perfume: Bitter almond oil is used occasionally in perfume but more often in medicines.

BITTER ORANGE OIL

In nature: This essential oil is expressed from the peel of the fruit of the bigarade orange tree.

In perfume: Chypre perfumes often contain bitter orange oil as part of their bouquet.

BLACK CURRANT BUD

In nature: This fragrant oil is obtained from the flower buds of the black currant bush.

In perfume: Black currant bud is a popular addition to many perfumes and appears as a top note in Delicious by Gale Haymen and as a heart note in Annick Goutal's Eau de Charlotte.

BLACK PEPPER

In nature: Black peppercorns are dried before their essential oil is distilled.

In perfume: Black pepper's warm and spicy notes blend well with sandalwood and frankincense. Guerlain's Héritage cologne for men has a spicy pepper heart note.

BOIS DE ROSE
In nature: Also called rosewood oil or linaloe, bois de rose is an essential oil with balsamic, mildly rose-scented notes. It is steam-distilled from a tree called rose fernelle.
In perfume: Bois de rose is often used in lilac and lily perfumes.

CARDAMOM
In nature: This spicy essential oil is distilled from the seeds of an East Indian herb in the ginger family.
In perfume: Its use dates back to ancient Egypt and is often used in floral and citrus perfumes. Examples of perfumes with cardamom are Lauder's Aramis for Men, where it is used as a middle note, and Byzance by Rochas where it is used as a top note.

CARNATION
In nature: This well-known flower is cultivated in the south of France.
In perfume: Carnation's spicy, clove-like odor lends a warm, sensuous note to a fragrance blend. White carnations are favored as their scent is the most robust. Examples of carnation-scented perfumes are Bellodgia (Caron) and L'Air du Temps (Ricci).

CASSIE
In nature: This oil is distilled from the *Acacia farnesiana* bush. The absolute made from the oil has a spicy, floral aroma.
In perfume: Cassie appears primarily in perfumes in the Oriental family and is a base note in Parfum Sacré by Caron.

CASTOREUM
In nature: Castoreum is a secretion produced by the beaver, and it was used to create leather or chypre notes. Only synthetic forms of this fixative are used today.
In perfume: Castoreum is found in base notes in such perfumes as Givenchy's Ysatis.

CEDARWOOD OIL

In nature: This essential oil is distilled from the American and Moroccan juniper cedar tree.

In perfume: Cedarwood oil is used as a base note for perfume and in men's cologne. In early times, its twigs and bark were used in incense. Magie Noire (Lancôme) has a rich cedarwood essence and Kenzo pour Homme has cedarwood base notes.

CINNAMON (also known as cassia)

In nature: This familiar baking spice comes from the dried bark, twigs, and buds of a tree or shrub which grows in Ceylon.

In perfume: Like many of the spicy fragrance ingredients, cinnamon can be used as a top, middle, or base note. For example, in Patou's Ma Liberté, cinnamon is a base note while in Karan's Chaos, it is a top note.

CITRONELLA

In nature: This pungent lemon-scented oil is extracted from grasses in Ceylon.

In perfume: Citronella is used primarily in candles as a mosquito repellent. It also appears as a top note in scented soaps and occasionally in perfumes.

CIVET

In nature: Civet is taken from the Ethiopian civet cat.

In perfume: Civet is a powerful fixative. The main supply comes from Africa, but a synthetic substitute is available. Venezia by Laura Biagiotti has civet as a prominent base note.

CLARY SAGE

In nature: The oil from this aromatic member of the mint family is distilled from blossoms of this sage.

In perfume: Clary sage tones a scent, adding a mellow, sweet note to fragrances, and is known to be an excellent fixative. The oil is an important addition to eau de cologne.

CLOVE BUD OIL

In nature: This essential oil is distilled from the dried flower buds of the clove tree.

In perfume: Clove bud oil is used to impart a sweet spicy note to both floral and spicy fragrances. It is used as a top note in Chanel's Coco.

COCONUT OIL

In nature: This white, semi-solid fat comes from the meat of the coconut.

In perfume: Coconut oil lathers well and is useful as a moisturizer or as a blending agent with other oils. It is liquid at room temperature.

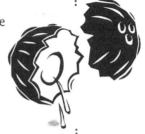

CORIANDER

In nature: This essential oil is steam-distilled from the seeds of the small, annual coriander plant.

In perfume: Coriander seeds were found in the tomb of King Tutankhamun. The chypre perfume Coriandré uses this spice as a top note.

COSTUS

In nature: The roots of this large plant, which grows in the Himalayas around Kashmir, render a fragrant oil.

In perfume: Costus oil smooths the violet note in a fragrance blend and imparts a warm, unique note to Oriental blends.

CYCLAMEN

In nature: This flower, which is a close cousin to the primrose, is native to the Alps.

In perfume: Cyclamen is used as a base note in Laura Ashley No. 1.

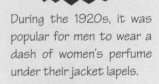

During the 1920s, it was popular for men to wear a dash of women's perfume under their jacket lapels.

EUGENOL

In nature: This is the main chemical in oil of cloves.

In perfume: Eugenol is also found in carnations, allspice, bay, cinnamon leaf, and patchouli, adding a spicy clove note to their aromas.

FRANGIPANI

In nature: This small, flowering tree from the American tropics was named after the sixteenth century Italian nobleman Muzio Frangipane.

In perfume: Leather gloves were once scented with this jasmine-like fragrance and known as "Frangipani gloves." This scent is a heart note in the lovely perfume Escada, by Margaret Ley.

FRANKINCENSE

In nature: This very fragrant gum resin, also called olibanum, has an ancient lineage and is one of the most famous scents in history. Frankincense comes from deciduous trees and shrubs in Somalia and south coastal Arabia. It has a sharp, sweet balsam odor when burned as incense and was commonly used in religious ceremonies.

In perfume: Frankincense is a wonderful fixative and is used as a base note in many perfumes.

FREESIA

In nature: These sweet-scented members of the iris family grow in Africa.

In perfume: The delicious scent of freesia has never been successfully extracted, so it is reproduced synthetically for perfume and is used as a heart or middle note. Antonia's Flowers (Antonia Bellanca) is primarily a freesia fragrance.

GALBANUM

In nature: This aromatic, bitter gum resin is derived from several Asian plants.

In perfume: Galbanum exudes a fresh, green, leaf-like smell and is used as a base note. It is also used in incense.

GARDENIA

In nature: These showy white flowers are found in the tropical regions of Europe.

In perfume: The rich and velvety odor of gardenia absolute is quite costly. Gardenia Passion by Annick Goutal is a pure gardenia scent.

GERANIUM

In nature: Although there are many different varieties of scented geraniums, rose geraniums and palma rose geraniums are the most commonly used in perfumery. But others, such as mint, lemon, nutmeg, apple, apricot, ginger, orange, and pineapple are also part of the perfumer's palette. They also dry well and are commonly used in fragrance crafting.

In perfume: The essential oil from scented geraniums is steam-distilled from the plant and appears as a middle note in Chopard's Casmir.

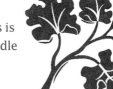

GINGER

In nature: The essential oil from this familiar spice is distilled from the rhizomes of the ginger plant.

In perfume: This warm, pungently spicy oil adds zest to Oriental and modern blends.

GUM

In nature: Many aromatic barks, twigs, and leaves produce resinous substances used in the perfume industry. Gums are often referred to as resins or balsams. Specific examples of gums used in perfume are styrax benzoin and gum benzoin.

In perfume: Gums are used as fixatives in the base notes of perfume.

GLYCERIN

In nature: When fats are mixed with lye to make soap, glycerin (or glycol) is a by-product.

In perfume: Glycerin is a wonderful skin moisturizer and is useful in prolonging shelf life in fragrance crafting. You will note its addition in several recipes in chapter 5.

GRAPEFRUIT

In nature: The essential oil is steam-distilled from the peel of this familiar fruit.

In perfume: The French call grapefruit "pamplemousse" and it is almost always used as a top note, adding piquancy to a blend. Tommy Hilfiger's tommy has a top note of grapefruit, as does Donna Karan's Tuscany per Donna.

HELIOTROPE

In nature: Heliotrope oil is derived from herbs or shrubs in the borage family and has a distinctive vanilla/almond aroma.

In perfume: This lovely, aromatic plant should be part of everyone's garden. Heliotrope appears as a heart note in Sun, Moon, Stars by Lagerfeld and as a base note in Chant d'Arômes by Guerlain.

HONEY

In nature: This familiar sweet substance manufactured by bees from the nectar of flowers is usually replaced by a synthetic in today's perfumery. The scent of honey is quite tenacious and was once used in Arabian perfumes.

In perfume: When used in perfume, a honey note is referred to as a miel note. It appears as a top note in Thierry Mugler's Angel and as a base note in White Linen by Lauder.

HONEYSUCKLE

In nature: This tropical shrub blooms by night, as daytime heat would cause too much evaporation for the flowers to survive.

In perfume: Middle notes are where this fragrance appears with its sweet, warm jasmine-like aroma. Byblos has a delicious honeysuckle note.

HYACINTH

In nature: Hyacinths are members of the lily family and possess a sweet, green aroma.

In perfume: The low yield of essential oil makes this a costly ingredient, so it is usually reproduced synthetically. Cristalle (Chanel), Gió (Armani), and Private Collection (Lauder) all contain prevalent heart notes of hyacinth.

JASMINE

In nature: It takes 12,000 pounds of flowers from the Asian jasmine shrub to produce two pounds of the oil absolute used in perfumery. Blossoms from the first flowering are gathered in July and August but the second flowering in October provides the most fragrant blooms. Jasmine must be picked before dawn or 20 percent of the fragrance will be lost.

In perfume: Jasmine's white petals produce an oil which is an ingredient in almost every fine perfume. Essence of jasmine is obtained through enfleurage as the flowers continue to create fragrance after they are picked.

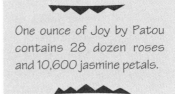

One ounce of Joy by Patou contains 28 dozen roses and 10,600 jasmine petals.

JOJOBA OIL

In nature: Jojoba oil is pressed from the seed kernels of an evergreen desert plant, producing a golden, naturally liquid wax. The vitamin E and minerals in jojoba oil soften skin, making it feel like silk.

In perfume: Jojoba oil is used as a carrier oil in fragrance crafting. By itself, it is good for inflamed skin or for mature skin needing nourishment. It is also used in the treatment of eczema and psoriasis. It is an excellent carrier oil for perfume because it will not turn rancid.

JONQUIL

In nature: This species of narcissus has been cultivated in the south of France since the eighteenth century for its essential oil.

In perfume: This is the perfumer's first choice from the narcissus family because it is the most fragrant. Jonquil is the middle note in Liz Claiborne perfume and in Vol de Nuit by Guerlain.

JUNIPER

In nature: This tree, which is a member of the cypress family, has a sweet honey and pine odor. Its oil is steam-distilled for use in perfumery.

In perfume: Juniper is used primarily in men's fragrances to add a woody note. It appears in Claiborne for Men.

LABDANUM

In nature: This gummy, sweet, honey-scented oleoresin is obtained from the rockrose.

In perfume: Labdanum is a valuable fixative which closely resembles the sperm whale's ambergris. Its central ingredient, ambrein, is used to manufacture synthetic ambers. Lagerfeld's KL rests on a base of labdanum.

LAVANDIN
In nature: This is a hybrid plant developed by crossing true lavender with spike or aspic lavender.
In perfume: It is used frequently in perfumery but cannot compare in fragrance to true lavender.

LAVENDER
In nature: The purple flowers and leaves of this aromatic plant have been used for perfumes and sachets for centuries. Five thousand tons of lavender flowers come from the south of France alone.
In perfume: Lavender oil is processed through steam distillation. It is a common ingredient in men's fragrances such as Le Male by Gaultier.

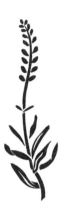

LEMONGRASS
In nature: Lemongrass comes from India and the Middle East. The oil is steam- or water-distilled.
In perfume: Lemongrass is used primarily in soaps or in bath salts.

LEMON OIL
In nature: This essential oil is expressed from the peel of the lemon.
In perfume: Lemon oil is used in top notes and imparts a refreshingly tangy scent. It is a top note in Balmain's famous Vent Vert. It is also an ingredient in 4711 Eau de Cologne, introduced to the world of fragrance in 1792.

LILAC
In nature: This well-loved shrub is native to Europe and is also known as syringa. It is a member of the olive family.
In perfume: Since the amount of oil extracted from the lilac is sparse, a perfumer is more likely to use synthetics to achieve a lilac scent. Design by Sebastian carries a heart note of lilac.

LILY

In nature: This essential oil comes from the Madonna lily or the Bourbon (Easter) lily and has been used in perfumery since ancient times.

In perfume: Many varieties of lily, including calla lilies, are used in perfumery. Cabotine (Grès) and Destiny (Miglin) both use lily as a heart note.

LILY OF THE VALLEY

In nature: The tiny, white, bell-like flowers of this low-growing plant provide one of the more familiar scents to perfumery.

In perfume: The fragrance of lily of the valley is extracted by volatile solvents as a concrete or absolute and has an exquisite fragrance. This scent is also known as muguet. Diorissimo (Dior) is a classic lily of the valley scent.

LIME OIL

In nature: The West Indian lime trees provide the fruit whose rind is used to obtain oil through expression or distillation.

In perfume: Lime oil is a popular top note and appears in fragrances such as Eau de Rochas and Royall Lime After Shave.

LINALOE OIL — SEE BOIS DE ROSE

MACE

In nature: Mace is the covering or net that surrounds the nutmeg.

In perfume: This pungent spice and essential oil provides an unusual top note in Clinique's Wrappings.

MAGNOLIA
In nature: The flowers of this evergreen tree bloom in the spring.
In perfume: Since magnolia flowers do not produce the oil necessary for perfume, their full-bodied scent is reproduced by a blend of rose, jasmine, neroli, and ylang-ylang oils. Lalique perfume has a heart note of magnolia.

MANDARIN
In nature: This small, spiny tree is native to southeastern Asia. Its oil is similar to that of sweet orange and is expressed from the fruit peel.
In perfume: Mandarin appears most often as a top note and is found in such compositions as Sung (Alfred Sung) and Amarige (Givenchy).

MARIGOLD
In nature: The showy red, orange, and maroon flowers of the genus *Tagetes* produce an oil with a fruity fragrance with apple-like overtones.
In perfume: Marigold is found as a heart note in Boucheron and Realm (Erox).

MELON
In nature: The scents of watermelon, honeydew, and cantaloupe are either steam-distilled or reproduced synthetically for use in perfume.
In perfume: Melon appears as a top note in 360° (Perry Ellis), Calyx (Prescriptives), and Elysium (Clarins).

MIGNONETTE
In nature: Mignonette produces dainty white flowers with a violet-like scent.
In perfumery: The oil is very powerful and only used in minute quantities as a heart note.

MIMOSA
In nature: The small yellow flowers of this warmth-loving tree are very fragrant, with sweet, waxy undertones.

In perfume: This floral absolute is extracted from the flowers by means of volatile solvents. Ralph Lauren's Lauren and Chanel's Coco contain mimosa.

MUSK

In nature: This penetrating aromatic is obtained from a sack in the abdomen of the male musk deer and is one of the most potent oils used in perfumery. Because of its scarcity and costliness, most musk is reproduced synthetically.

In perfume: Musk is an excellent and widely used fixative. Must de Cartier has a base note of musk.

MYRRH

In nature: This pungent aromatic appears as tears of resin on the bark of trees in northern Africa and Arabia.

In perfume: Myrrh is used in base notes as a fixative in perfumes such as DNA by Bijan and Opium by St. Laurent.

NARCISSUS

In nature: The oil of these daffodils is extracted with volatile solvents or through enfleurage. The yellow and white flowers emit a heady fragrance that is expensive and highly valued by perfumers.

In perfume: Narcissus is most commonly used as a heart note and appears in fragrances such as Chloé Narcisse by Lagerfeld, Gale Haymen's Delicious, and Destiny by Marilyn Miglin.

NEROLI OIL

In nature: This pale yellow, essential oil is steam-distilled from orange blossoms. It takes one ton of blossoms to produce two pounds of neroli oil.

In perfume: Neroli oil appears as both a top and middle note. For example, it is a top note in Paloma Picasso perfume and a middle note in Grey Flannel by Geoffrey Beene.

NIGHT-SCENTED STOCK

In nature: These pink and purple night-blooming flowers produce a sweet, penetrating oil.

In perfume: This flower is used as a middle note in perfumery.

NUTMEG

In nature: Nutmeg is the fruit of an evergreen tree native to the Indonesian islands.

In perfume: Nutmeg is often used in lavender water, is a significant scent in Patou's Ma Liberté, a top note in Ivoire (Balmain), and a heart note in Todd Oldham perfume.

OAKMOSS

In nature: Oakmoss is actually the resin of several different lichens which grow on oak trees.

In perfume: This fragrance is often used in chypre and fougère blends. It's an excellent fixative imparting earthy and woody notes to a perfume and is a principal ingredient in one-third of all men's and women's fragrances.

OPOPONAX

In nature: This resin shares the same genus as myrrh.

In perfume: Opoponax is an excellent fixative with sweet, woody undertones. It is used as a replacement for many of the perfume ingredients that come from animals. It is found in the base notes of Oscar de la Renta and Nicole Miller perfumes.

ORANGE BLOSSOM

In nature: A flowering shrub produces these delicate blossoms.

In perfume: Orange blossoms are most often used as heart notes and are a popular ingredient in perfumes such as Jardins de Bagatelle (Guerlain).

ORANGEFLOWER WATER

In nature: The water left behind when orange blossoms are distilled to make neroli oil has a wonderful aroma. Orangeflower water was once referred to as sweet water.

In perfume: Strictly speaking, orangeflower water is not used in perfumery, but it works wonderfully as a splash all by itself. It is included in the recipe for Florida Water on page 79.

ORRIS

In nature: Orris is made from the dried rhizomes of certain iris species.

In perfume: Orris is a superb fixative with a violet scent. Brousseau's Ombre Rose and Samsara by Guerlain both contain orris oil.

OSMANTHUS
In nature: This jasminelike fragrance, which is underlined with plum and raisin notes, comes from the flowers of an evergreen tree growing in China and Japan.
In perfume: The essence of osmanthus is found in 1000 de Jean Patou and Venezia by Laura Biagiotti.

PALMA ROSE OIL
In nature: This fragrance ingredient is steam-distilled from the leaves of the rose geranium.
In perfume: Used extensively in perfume, palma rose oil is always a lovely addition to rose fragrance blends.

PATCHOULI
In nature: This essential oil is steam-distilled from the leaves of a shrubby mint native to India.
In perfume: Patchouli possesses powerful fixative properties. Its musty, earthy scent is a base note in one-third of women's and half of men's fragrances. Antilope (Weil) uses patchouli as a base note. Look for patchouli plants in the herb section of your garden center. They are easily dried for use in potpourri.

PEACH
In nature: The essence of peach can be distilled from the juice of this fruit, but perfumers usually use a synthetic peach ingredient because it is stronger.
In perfume: Guerlain's Mitsouko was the first perfume to use peach as a smooth, mellow top note. Ellen Tracy perfume and Arden's Sunflowers also have peach notes.

PEAR
In nature: Perfumers use a synthetic reproduction of the scent of this familiar fruit.
In perfume: There are pear notes in Smalto Donna by Francesco Smalto and Il Bacio by Borghese has a lovely pear essence as one its fruity top notes.

PENNYROYAL

In nature: When the leaves of this herb are steam-distilled, they produce a fragrant, minty oil.

In perfume: Pennyroyal is not used in perfumery but it is a great additive to pet shampoos because of its wonderful aroma and because it is a good flea repellent.

PEPPERMINT

In nature: This is the best-known member of the mint family. Its oil is used occasionally in perfumery, but its primary use is in pharmaceuticals.

In perfume: Peppermint does form one of the top notes of Romà by Biagiotti. The dried leaves of this plant are a wonderful addition to potpourri and insect repellent blends. Mice don't like the scent of peppermint either.

PETITGRAIN

In nature: The bitter orange trees of southern France are a source of three fragrance ingredients: Neroli oil is distilled from the tree's flowers with orangeflower water as a by-product, while petitgrain is distilled from the tree's leaves and twigs.

In perfume: Petitgrain imparts a mellow note to perfume and is often paired with lemon or orange. Eau d'Hermès has petitgrain as a base note although it's more often used as a top note.

PINE NEEDLE OIL

In nature: This oil is steam-distilled from the needles, twigs, and stems of dwarf and Scotch pines.

In perfume: This is used primarily in green or woody compositions. Pino Silvestre by Classic Fragrances, Ltd., is a pine-scented men's cologne.

PINEAPPLE

In nature: Oil from this tropical fruit is distilled from its juice.

In perfume: Perfumers use pineapple oil or produce this scent synthetically. Pineapple notes can be found in C'est la Vie by Lacroix, and the unisex fragrance cK one by Calvin Klein.

PLUM

In nature: This familiar purple fruit does not yield oil for use in the perfume industry.

In perfume: The fruity note of the mirabelle plum is achieved synthetically in modern perfumery. Several examples of perfumes with plum or mirabelle notes are Chant d'Arômes by Guerlain, Escape by Calvin Klein, and Y by St. Laurent.

RASPBERRY

In nature: These delicious red berries grow on bushes but the essence is reproduced synthetically for use in perfume.

In perfume: Estée (Estée Lauder) employs raspberry as a top note.

RESIN

In nature: The many gums derived from trees, in particular pine and other evergreens, are called resins in perfumery.

In perfume: Resins are commonly used as fixatives.

RESINOIDS

In nature: These substances are extracts of gums, balsams, and orris roots that contain resinous materials.

In perfume: Resinoids are used as fixatives.

RONDELETIA

In nature: The rondeletia shrub is native to Cuba and Mexico.

In perfume: This scent does not come directly from a natural source. In perfumery, rondeletia is made with a combination of lavender and cloves.

ROSE BULGARE

In nature: The damask rose *(Rosa damascena)* is cultivated in Bulgaria's Valley of the Roses and in Turkey. Damask roses were introduced to Europe by Crusaders. Rose bulgare is considered the finest rose fragrance in the world.

In perfume: To extract a pound of oil, 4,000 pounds of roses are needed. Rose oil is used in 82 percent of women's and 12 percent of all men's fragrances. There are nearly 20 different rose scents, among them myrrh-, clove-, fruity-, and musk-scented varieties. Rose bulgare is a primary ingredient in Joy

(Patou). Because of the expense of rose bulgare, its scent is reproduced synthetically for home fragrance crafting.

ROSE DE MAI

In nature: This flower, often called the cabbage rose *(Rosa centifolia)*, blooms only in May, hence its name. Grown primarily in the south of France, it has a sweet odor, is somewhat lighter than Bulgarian rose, and is half the price. It's also referred to as the blue rose.

In perfume: Rose de Mai is the heart note in Bal à Versailles (Jean Despres), Safari (Ralph Lauren), Chanel No. 19 (Chanel), and Oscar de la Renta perfume.

ROSEMARY

In nature: This herb thrives along the coast of the Mediterranean Sea. Its name means "dew of the sea." Its camphor and lavender-like fragrance is distilled from the leaves and flowers.

In perfume: Rosemary oil is a major ingredient in Hungary water, one of the first perfumes ever created. It appears as a base note in Guerlain's Eau de Cologne Impèriale and is often coupled with lavender in men's colognes such as Egoïste Platinum (Chanel), and Cool Water (Davidoff).

ROSEWATER

In nature: The floral essences of damask and centifolia roses are used in rosewater.

In perfume: While it is not now used in commercial perfumery, this beloved sweet water was discovered by the Arabs in the ninth century and introduced to Europe via Spain in the tenth century. It is often an ingredient in home fragrance crafting, being a wonderful toner for all skin types, and an excellent hand lotion when mixed with glycerin.

SANDALWOOD

In nature: The best sandalwood comes from parasitic trees growing in Mysore, India, and has a warm, woodsy aroma.

In perfumery: Sandalwood is an excellent fixative and appears as a base note in over half of the women's and one-third of the men's perfumes. Such a large quantity of sandalwood is used in

Guerlain's Samsara that the company bought its own plantation in India. Caswell-Massey and Crabtree & Evelyn both have single note sandalwood scents that are wonderful.

SIBERIAN FIR
In nature: This oil is distilled from the fresh leaves of the Siberian fir.
In perfume: This oil is used in woody blends.

STAR ANISE
In nature: Found in China, this anise-scented fruit is from a large, evergreen tree. Its yellow flowers are followed by the appearance of eight-pointed, star-shaped fruit containing brown seeds within the points of the star.
In perfume: Star anise is a spicy top note in Jean-Paul Gaultier perfume.

STEPHANOTIS
In nature: This strongly scented flowering vine, with a fragrance of jasmine and tuberose, is native to the tropical regions of Europe. It is a very popular addition to wedding bouquets. Caswell-Massey carries a wonderful stephanotis oil for fragrance crafting. (See the Source Guide on page 153).
In perfume: Nocturnes by Caron has a heart note of stephanotis.

STYRAX
In nature: Styrax, or storax as it is sometimes called, is a balsam reminiscent of vanilla with strong fixative qualities.
In perfume: This ingredient is commonly used as a base note. When used sparingly, its bouquet resembles a combination of hyacinth, jonquil, and tuberose. K de Krizia has a base note of styrax.

SWEET ALMOND OIL
In nature: This colorless to pale yellow, scentless carrier oil is expressed from the seeds of sweet almonds.
In perfume: Sweet almond oil benefits all skin types and has excellent penetrating qualities. It is a wonderful carrier oil for fragrance compounds to be used in the bath or for massage.

SWEET ORANGE

In nature: This essential oil is distilled from the peel of the fruit from the sweet orange tree.

In perfume: Sweet orange is used in flavorings as well as in citrus blend perfumes, and in eau de colognes. It appears as a heart note in Tendre Poison.

SWEET PEA

In nature: The essential oil of this flowering vine is extracted through enfleurage and has the fragrance of hyacinth, orange blossom, vanilla, and a touch of rose.

In perfume: Old-fashioned sweet peas have an unforgettable scent. Floret by Antonia Bellanca is an excellent example of the fragrance of a bouquet of sweet peas.

TANGERINE

In nature: This oil is expressed from the fruit's peel.

In perfume: Tangerine provides a crisp orange fragrance in the top notes of Dolce and Gabbana perfume. The men's fragrance Boss Elements by Hugo Boss has a top note of tangerine.

THYME

In nature: The oil is distilled from the leaves of this herb. Perfumery uses several species of thyme including lemon thyme and also a spicy variety.

In perfume: This herbal essential oil combines nicely with lavender oil to produce an herbal, green note in perfumery. Safari for Men (Lauren) has a middle note of thyme.

TONKA BEAN

In nature: The beans of the American tonka tree yield an oil which is sometimes used as a substitute for vanilla. Tonka also has a new-mown hay scent to it because it contains coumarin.

In perfume: It is used as a base note and popular with perfumers, appearing in Le Dix by Balenciaga, Panthère by Cartier, and White Linen by Estée Lauder. It is also chopped up and added to potpourri to impart a vanilla-like fixative to the overall scent.

TUBEROSE

In nature: Tuberose is a member of the lily family and possesses a rich, sensuous fragrance. A few blooms will scent an entire room.

In perfume: Tuberose is one of the most expensive essential oils and is obtained through enfleurage. Gardenia, narcissus, hyacinth, and jonquil are enhanced by the addition of tuberose. Blonde by Versace, Fracas by Piguet, and Chloé by Lagerfeld are beautiful examples of perfumes with tuberose.

TURKEY RED OIL

In nature: This oil is expressed from the castor oil bean. Nowadays, turkey red oil is put through a process through which it becomes sulfonated.

In perfume: This is the only oil that mixes with and disperses in water, making it a wonderful carrier oil for fragrant bath products made in home fragrance crafting.

VANILLA

In nature: This familiar fragrance is obtained from the fruit or seeds of a climbing orchid native to Madagascar.

In perfume: Vanilla adds richness and depth to many sweet floral or amber bases. Strong vanilla notes can be found in Shalimar by Guerlain, Angel by Thierry Mugler, and Casmir by Chopard.

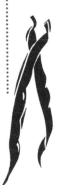

VANILLIN

In nature: This crystalline aldehyde is extracted from vanilla pods or created synthetically.

In perfume: Vanillin is a valued fixative in perfumery but lacks the full-bodied quality of vanilla.

VERBENA

In nature: The essential oil is distilled from the leaves of lemon verbena.

In perfume: This clean, fresh, lemon scent is used in soaps and sometimes in perfumes, especially citrus formulas.

VETIVER

In nature: This essential oil is distilled from the rhizomes of khus-khus grass grown in India.

In perfume: Vetiver has an earthy, woodsy aroma and is one of the finest fixatives known. Knowing by Estée Lauder, a chypre perfume, uses vetiver as a base note. In fact, most chypre perfumes use vetiver. It complements jasmine and sandalwood.

VIOLET

In nature: This highly fragrant essential oil is obtained from the flowers of the Parma and the Victoria violets through enfleurage. It was a favorite scent in the Victorian era. A second essential oil, violet leaf, adds an earthy, herbaceous note to perfumes.

In perfume: Since violet absolute is very costly, this fragrance is often made synthetically on an ionone base with the addition of natural violet extract. Fragrances with violet notes are Fleurs de Rocaille by Caron, Après L'Ondée by Guerlain, and L'Interdit by Givenchy. It is also found in Grey Flannel by Grès/Geoffrey Beene.

WATER LILY

In nature: This flower yields an essential oil.

In perfume: The floral fragrance 360° by Perry Ellis has a heart note of water lily.

WHEAT GERM OIL

In nature: This wonderful carrier oil is pressed from the heart of wheat. It contains the skin-nourishing properties of vitamin E, along with lecithin and vitamins A and D.

In perfume: Wheat germ oil is especially good for use on mature skin and on stretch marks. It is often used as an anti-bacterial agent in cosmetic preparations.

YLANG-YLANG

In nature: The name means "flower of flowers" and the oil comes from a tree native to Madagascar and the Phillippines.

In perfume: This flower oil is rich, sweetly balsamic, and jasminelike. It adds a lift to oriental types of perfume and blends well with violet and jasmine. There are many perfumes made with ylang-ylang, including Dilys by Laura Ashley, Jardins de Bagatelle by Guerlain, and Jean-Paul Gaultier. Ylang-ylang is wonderful to use in fragrance crafting, and as a single note fragrance.

CHAPTER 3

BUILDING YOUR FRAGRANCE PROFILE

A fragrance wardrobe is an extension of your personal expression. There are several factors to consider as you build your fragrance wardrobe — your personality, the climate you live in, your skin type, diet, and body chemistry. And as you make your daily decisions about what fragrance to wear, you'll factor in such information as the time of day, occasion, season and, of course, personal preference.

To help you decide what to include in your fragrance wardrobe, this chapter includes a quiz to determine your fragrance preferences, several fragrance profiles, and lots of advice about choosing and wearing perfumes.

QUIZ #1

One of the factors governing your perfume selection is how well and how long scent lingers on your skin. This first quiz will help you determine how well fragrances last on you. Your answers will determine whether you should steer yourself towards heavier fragrances, whether cologne is a better choice for you than perfume, or whether a light splash of rosewater is all you need to carry you through the day.

1. Is your hair color
a) Brown? b) Blond? c) Red?

2. Is your skin type
a) Oily? b) Normal? c) Dry?

3. Do you take birth control or other hormonal medications?
   a) Yes   b) No

4. Do you take other prescription medications?
   a) Yes   b) No

5. Is your skin tone
   a) Dark?   b) Medium?   c) Fair?

6. Do you live in a hot climate?
   a) Yes   b) Variable   c) No

7. Do you engage in a lot of strenuous activities and
   exercise?
   a) Yes   b) Sometimes   c) No

8. Do you eat fruit every day?
   a) Yes   b) No

9. Do you eat a lot of spicy foods?
   a) Yes   b) No

10. Do you have a high or low fat diet?
   a) High   b) Low

11. Are you an extrovert or an introvert?
   a) Extrovert   b) Introvert

12. Do you perspire a lot?
   a) Yes   b) No

Rating Your Answers
(add up numbers next to your answer)

1. a) 1	b) 2	c) 3		**7.** a) 3	b) 2	c) 1
2. a) 1	b) 2	c) 3		**8.** a) 3	b) 1	
3. a) 3	b) 1			**9.** a) 3	b) 1	
4. a) 3	b) 1			**10.** a) 3	b) 1	
5. a) 1	b) 2	c) 3		**11.** a) 3	b) 1	
6. a) 3	b) 2	c) 1		**12.** a) 3	b) 1	

Add up your score:

◆ 12–15 points: scent lasts well on you

◉ 15–22 points: at times your scent fades sooner than it
should

◆ 23–35 points: you definitely have a problem with your fragrance lasting

If fragrance is more pronounced on you, consider using
lighter scents such as citrus, oceanic, or lighter florals. Instead
of Eau de Parfum use Eau de Cologne, especially if you are not
wearing one of the lighter scents. If your scent fades sooner
than it should, try heavier scents or layering (as described on
page 62). If you are constantly re-applying your fragrance try
eau de parfum, creams or solid perfumes, layering, and oriental or floriental blends, which have slower evaporation rates.

Every person is an individual and has her own set of miti-
gating factors which affect how long a perfume will last and
how the fragrance develops on her. That is why it's important
to try a fragrance several times before purchasing it. When you
are crafting scents on your own, always write down your formulas and initially make small amounts until you discover your
fragrance preferences.

QUIZ #2

Our second quiz will help you determine what families of
fragrance best suit your personality. Once you have this information, move on to the fragrance profile section that follows.

Now let's have some fun imagining and imaging. Keep in
mind that aromas and fond memories walk hand in hand.

Colors (Which appeals to you most?)

A nature colors

B pastels

C naturals and deep tones

D southwest colors

E the colors of sunsets and moonlight

F rich tones and creamy ivory

G black, white, and red

H rainbow hues and deep green

I jewel tones

Aromas (Which appeals to you most?)

A fresh air, seaspray, citrus fruits

B old English roses, walking through a flower shop, scented candles

C cinnamon, ginger, nutmeg, lichens, and moss

D a walk through the woods, linens drying in the breeze

E apple pie, birthday cake, fresh peaches, violets

F incense, gardenias, and night-blooming jasmine

G blackberries, fragrant wood burning, lilies, narcissus

H freshly mown grass, juicy oranges, hyacinths, ocean air

I raspberries, tuberose, old books, leather

Activities (Which appeals to you most?)

A outdoor and water sports, horseback riding, hiking

B writing poems, gardening, making gifts for family and friends

C scuba diving, innovative cooking, chess

D working out at the gym, parties, competitive sports

E collecting beautiful things, Victoriana, tea parties in the rose garden, carousel rides

F shopping, decorating, gourmet dining, island hopping

G seminars, art galleries, French cuisine

H entertaining, friendships, volunteer work, potluck suppers, letter writing

I museums, European vacations, polo, old houses, concerts

Music (Which appeals to you most?)

A mood music, nature tapes

B Vivaldi, songs with a message, Rachmaninoff

C good old rock and roll

D jazz and the newest dance music

E show tunes, love songs

F classical and John Tesh concerts

G opera

H popular music

I piano and violin concertos

Entertainment (Which appeals to you most?)

A picnics in the meadow, canoe rides, visiting the zoo

B art and craft shows, visiting a teahouse, reading in a hammock

C coffee houses, unusual cuisine, visiting the local playhouse

D dancing the night away, jumping in the pool at midnight, good conversation

E candlelight dinners, dancing in the moonlight, bubble baths

F a relaxing massage at the spa, traveling to new places, dining alfresco

G going to the theatre and the ballet, vintage wines, drinking champagne

H making new friends and cherishing old ones, ice cream socials, going to the circus

I garden tours and flower shows, visiting designer houses, haute cuisine

If your answers were mostly:	Then You Prefer:
A	Citrus, oceanic, and marine scents
B	Floral bouquets and single floral scents
C	Spicy and chypre blends
D	Fresh, spicy florals, woodsy-mossy chypres
E	Fresh and fruity florals
F	Floriental, oriental, amber notes
G	Modern aldehydic scents that sparkle, florientals
H	Green, fruity, and marine scents
I	Oriental, modern, florientals

Remember, you will probably find several scent families that appeal to you. This quiz should help to aim you in the right direction and give you some suggestions while you are pursuing a fragrance wardrobe and crafting your own favorite medley.

FRAGRANCE PROFILES

Please be aware that several of the following profiles may appeal to you — and that's the way it should be. We are all complex individuals and will probably find portions of several profiles that appeal to us. Given the long history of perfume and all the scents available now, it's no surprise that building a fragrance wardrobe means weighing many factors as we consider our choices.

For example, many of us love sports, but that might mean a quiet game of croquet, hiking the Appalachian Trail, a vigorous game of tennis, or inline skating on a Sunday afternoon. Your love of eating out may be picnics, while to someone else it could be dining on exquisite French cuisine. Part of your life may be devoted to business, part to homemaking, and part to community service. There may be different scents appropriate for each of these sides of your life. In other words, when building a fragrance profile, explore your whole world and all of the facets of your personality.

The profiles are written with images to appeal to your sense of touch, color, and taste as well as smell. Please keep in mind as you read them that the fruits and spirits are mentioned for their fragrances, not necessarily as a reflection of your favorites to eat.

SPORTS AND OUTDOOR LOVER

Image: Sailing on azure seas under a brilliant sun. Munching crisp apples by a lake covered in water lilies. A nest of robin's eggs in a green, leafy tree. The scent of linens drying in the fresh air.

Flowers, fruits, and spirits: Hyacinth, water lilies, verbena, Granny Smith apples, mineral water, and calvados

Colors: Robin's egg blue, butter yellow, fresh lime, apricot

Gemstones: Peridot, aquamarine

Suggested fragrance families: Citrus; oceanic

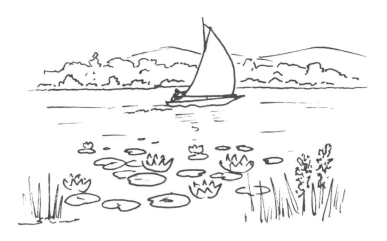

Suggested perfumes

Women

Acqua di Giô (Giorgio Armani)
Cristalle (Chanel)
Dalissimo (Salvador Dali)
Dune (Dior)
Fleur d'Eau (Rochas)
Giorgio Aire (Giorgio Beverly
    Hills)
Jill Sander #4 (Jill Sander)
L'Eau d'Issey (Issey Miyake)
Polo Sport for Women (Ralph
    Lauren)
Sunflowers (Arden)

Men

America for Men (Perry Ellis)
Eau d'Hadrien (Annick Goutal)
Impériale (Guerlain)
Lacoste (Patou)

Teenagers/Female

Citrus (Crabtree & Evelyn)
Day (The Gap, Inc.)
Earth (The Gap, Inc.)
Ocean Dreams (Giorgio Beverly
    Hills)
Sunny Sky (Avon)

Teenagers/Male

Polo Sport (Ralph Lauren)
tommy (Tommy Hilfiger)

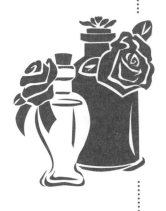

DREAMER

Images: Bouquets of fresh flowers scenting the air. Roses releasing their perfume as honeybees whirl about. Sweet, juicy melons. Blue, lavender, and pink lilacs blooming over a porch railing as you rock in the warmth of a summer day.

Flowers, fruits, and spirits: Stephanotis, orange blossoms, sweetheart roses, honeydew melon, and Midori liqueur

Colors: Blushing pink, misty blue, mint, lilac

Gemstones: Pink, green, and watermelon tourmalines

Suggested scent families: Floral blends; single florals

Suggested perfumes

Women

*Antonia's Flowers (Antonia
    Bellanca)
Curve (Liz Claiborne)
Destiny (Marilyn Miglin)
Diorissimo (Dior)
Eternity (Calvin Klein)
Fleurs de Rocaille (Caron)
Fracas (Piguet)
Jardins de Bagatelle (Guerlain)
Narcisse Noir (Caron)
360° (Perry Ellis)
    suitable for sport wear

Men

Cool Water (Davidoff)
English Lavender (Yardley)
Eternity for Men (Calvin Klein)
YSL Pour Hommes (Yves St.
    Laurent)

Teenagers/Female

Anaïs Anaïs (Cacheral)
Cherry Vanilla (Shiara)
Comfort Scents (Avon)
Dream (The Gap, Inc.)

Teenagers/Male

Cool Water (Davidoff)
Eternity for Men (Calvin Klein)

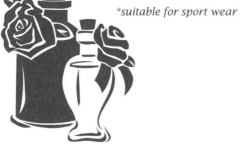

INDEPENDENT AND UNCONVENTIONAL

Images: A mossy glen, secluded, filled with ferns and wood-land flora. Lichen-covered stones beside a crystal stream. At home, spiced cider by a crackling fire of aromatic cedarwood.
Flowers, fruits, and spirits: Carnations, chrysanthemums, poppies, kiwi, starfruit, Pernod
Colors: Camel, aubergine, moss, acorn
Gemstones: Smoky topaz, amber, carnelian
Suggested scent families: Spicy; chypre

Suggested perfumes

Women

Aromatics Elixir (Clinique)
Cabochard (Grès)
Charlie (Revlon)
Coriandre (Couturier)
*Cristalle (Chanel)
First (Van Cleef & Arpels)
KL (Lagerfeld)
Ma Liberté (Patou)
Suitable for sport wear

Men

Boucheron Pour Homme
   (Boucheron)
Eau Savage (Dior)
Monsieur Givenchy (Givenchy)
Nightflight (Joop!)
Salvador (Salvador Dali)
Tuscany (Aramis)

Teenagers/Unisex scents

cK be (Calvin Klein)
cK one (Calvin Klein)
Paco (Paco Rabanne)

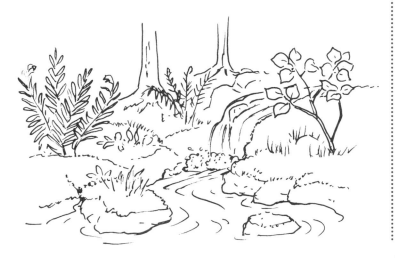

OUTGOING, SOCIABLE, AND ENERGETIC

Images: An herb garden filled with tantalizing scents and tastes. Lavender spikes perfuming the paths with their delicious, spicy aroma. Strawberries and cream.

Flowers, fruits, and spirits: Lavender, balsam, scented geraniums, strawberries, and Fraises des Bois liqueur

Colors: Sunset, teal, caramel, hunter green

Gemstones: Coral, jade, malachite

Suggested scent families: Fresh and spicy florals; woodsy-mossy chypres

Suggested perfumes

Women

*America for Women (Perry Ellis)
Chanel No. 19 (Chanel)
Dolce Vita (Dior)
Femme (Rochas)
Halston (Halston)
Miss Dior (Dior)
Paloma Picasso (Paloma Picasso)
Parfum d'Eté (Kenzo)
Private Collection (Estée Lauder)
Safari (Ralph Lauren)
Suitable for sport wear

Men

Davidoff (Davidoff)
Drakkar (La Roche)
Escada for Men (Adipar)
Monsieur Lanvin (Lanvin)
Royal Copenhagen Classic
   (Tsumura)

Teenagers/Female

Calyx (Prescriptives)
Giorgio Aire (Giorgio Beverly
   Hills)
tommy girl (Tommy Hilfinger)

Teenagers/Male

cK one (Calvin Klein)
Drakkar (La Roche)
Polo (Ralph Lauren)

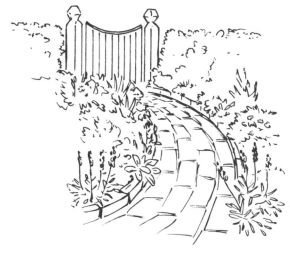

ROMANTIC

Images: A rock garden of violets and lilies of the valley. Delicate sweet peas climbing a trellis. Tea and petit fours, sunwarmed peaches and sparkling champagne in crystal flutes.

Flowers, fruits, and spirits: Sweet peas, lily of the valley, violets, peaches in champagne

Colors: Rose, periwinkle, celadon, peach, ivory

Gemstones: Amethyst, tanzanite

Suggested scent families: Fresh and fruity florals

Suggested perfumes

Women

Beautiful (Estée Lauder)
Champs Elysée (Guerlain)
Chanel No. 22 (Chanel)
Eternity (Calvin Klein)
Evelyn (Crabtree & Evelyn)
*Floret (Antonia Bellanca)
*Gieffeffe (Gianfranco Ferre)
Hanae Mori (Cosmetique et Parfum, Intn.)
L'Air du Temps (Nina Ricci)
Lalique (Lalique)
Laura Ashley No. 1 (Laura Ashley)
Nicole Miller (Nicole Miller)
No Regrets (Alexandra de Markoff)
Paris YSL (Yves St. Laurent)
So Pretty de Cartier (Cartier)
*Suitable for sport wear

Men

Eau de Givenchy (Givenchy)
Habit Rouge (Guerlain)
JHL (Lauder/Aramis)
Photo (Lagerfeld)
Wings for Men (Giorgio Beverly Hills)

Teenagers/Female

Chanel No. 22 (Chanel)
Jessica McClintock (Jessica McClintock)
True Love (Elizabeth Arden)
Vanilla (The Body Shop)

Teenagers/Male

HUGO (Proctor & Gamble)
Obsession (Calvin Klein)
Polo (Ralph Lauren)

SENSUAL, SELF-ASSURED, FASHIONABLE

Images: The enveloping scents of tuberose and gardenias filling the velvet night. Mellow pears, the smells of autumn, candlelight. Ruby Cabernet swirling in a goblet accompanied by foie gras and truffles.

Flowers, fruits, and spirits: Gardenia, heliotrope, tuberose, pears in Poire William brandy

Colors: Burgundy, plum, cream, jade

Gemstones: Ruby, garnet

Suggested scent families: Floriental; oriental; fruity

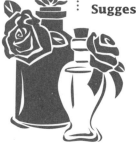

Suggested perfumes

Women	Men
*Aire de Samsara (Guerlain)	Equipage (Hermès)
Casmir (Chopard)	Kenzo Pour Homme (Kenzo)
Chloé (Lagerfeld)	Paco Rabanne (Paco Rabanne)
*Dalissimo (Salvador Dali)	Realm for Men (Erox Corp.)
Escada (Adipar)	XS (Paco Rabanne)
Grand Amour (Annick Goutal)	
Il Bacio (Marcella Borghese)	
L'Heure Bleu (Guerlain)	
Nahema (Guerlain)	
Obsession (Calvin Klein)	
Opium (Yves St. Laurent)	
Realm (Erox Corp.)	
Shalimar (Guerlain)	
Venezia (Laura Biagiotti)	
Youth Dew (Estée Lauder)	

Suitable for sport wear

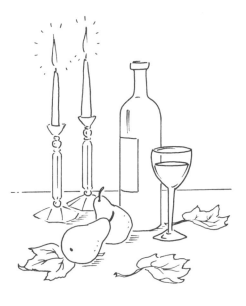

CAREER-ORIENTED

Images: Creamy calla lilies reflected in silver mirrors. Black-berries, plump and juicy atop white chocolate mousse. Kir Royale shimmering like jewels. Sandalwood carvings on a rose-wood desk alight with vanilla-scented candles.

Flowers, fruits, and spirits: Calla lily, damask rose, peonies, blackberries, Kir Royale

Colors: Black, red, beige

Gemstones: Pearls, jet

Suggested scent families: Modern; florientals

Suggested perfumes

Women	Men
Allure (Chanel)	Aramis (Aramis)
Bal à Versailles (Desprez)	Bulgari Pour Homme (Bulgari)
Boucheron (Boucheron)	Drakkar Noire (La Roche)
Coco (Chanel)	Grey Flannel (Geoffrey Beene)
Je Reviens (Worth)	Kouros (Yves St. Laurent)
Joy (Patou)	Smalto (Smalto)
Madame Rochas (Rochas)	
Nocturnes (Caron)	
Panthère (Cartier)	
Realities (Liz Claiborne)	
Rive Gauche (Yves St. Laurent)	
Spellbound (Estée Lauder)	
*White Linen Breeze (Estée Lauder)	

*Suitable for sport wear

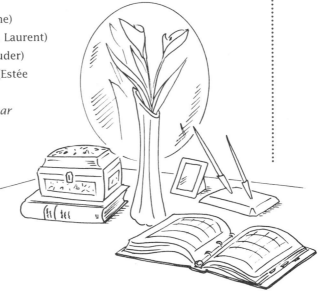

ELEGANT, FORMAL

Images: Mimosa blossoms dance in the wind, lacing the veranda with sweet perfume. Tea roses sway in a cobalt vase, spreading scents of lemon, myrrh, and raspberry. Peach melbas rest on a dessert table with delicate glasses of fragrant Chambord liqueur.
Flowers, fruits, and spirits: Tea rose, jasmine, mimosa, raspberries, Chambord liqueur
Colors: Royal blue, deep rose, purple, pearl grey
Gemstones: Sapphire, lapis lazuli
Suggested scent families: Oriental; floriental; modern

Suggested perfumes

Women

Arpège (Lanvin)
Bellodgia (Caron)
Blonde (Versace)
Byzance (Rochas)
*Escada Sport Feeling Free
   (Adipar)
5th Avenue (Elizabeth Arden)
Jean Paul Gaultier (Jean Paul
   Gaultier)
Kashaya (Kenzo)
L'Interdit (Givenchy)
1000 De Jean Patou (Patou)
Oscar de la Renta (Oscar de la
   Renta)
Samsara (Guerlain)
Suitable for sport wear

Men

Bulgari Pour Homme (Bulgari)
Egoïste Platinum (Chanel)
Givenchy (Givenchy)
Gucci Nobile (Gucci)
Van Cleef & Arpels (Van Cleef &
   Arpels)

NATURAL CHARM,
LOVES TO ENTERTAIN, EXTROVERT

Images: A wildflower meadow filled with the sweet scent of honeysuckle. Picnicking by a pond, watching a beaver build its dam. Enjoying a juicy orange while basking in the warmth of summer. Napping on grandma's quilt spread upon the verdant, scented grass.

Flowers, fruits, and spirits: Freesia, lilacs, honeysuckle, mandarin oranges, Grand Marnier liqueur

Colors: Forest, lavender, pearl, rose, azure

Gemstones: Emeralds, malachite, moonstone

Suggested scent families: Green; fruity; marine

Suggested perfumes

Women

Angel (Thierry Mugler)
Bulgari (Bulgari)
Byblos (Byblos)
Calèche (Hermès)
Chanel No. 5 (Chanel)
Dolce Vita (Dior)
Escape (Calvin Klein)
Giŏ (Giorgio Armani)
Je Reviens (Worth)
Lauren (Ralph Lauren)
*Pleasures (Estée Lauder)
Trésor (Lancôme)

Suitable for sport wear

Men

Bijan for Men (Bijan)
Giorgio Beverly Hills
    (Giorgio Beverly Hills)
Gucci Pour Homme (Gucci)
Pino Silvestre (Vidal)
Safari (Ralph Lauren)

Teenagers/Female

Clean Cotton (Avon)
Gieffeffe (Gianfranco Ferre)
Grass (The Gap, Inc.)
Heaven (The Gap, Inc.)

Teenagers/Male

Canoe Sport (Renaissance
    Cosmetics)
New West for Him (Aramis)

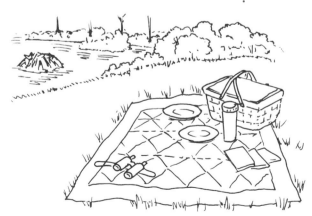

HOW (EXACTLY) TO WEAR PERFUME

The proper application of scent begins with your morning shower. Always use a matching scented soap or one that is scentless, as deodorant soap can eradicate or weaken your fragrance. Then apply layers of fragrance starting with a lotion or cream, followed by dusting powder then eau de parfum, toilet water, or cologne. Body creams, as opposed to lotions, have a much higher concentration of perfume oils and because of their cream base, will often outlast perfume. In addition, their emollients are kind to the skin.

Remember, fragrance rises, so be sure to put some behind your knees as on well as your other favorite pulse points — ear lobes, throat, the bend in your elbow, wrist, and between your breasts. Do not rub perfume into the skin as this damages the perfume's molecular structure, and don't spray perfume in your hair unless it is freshly washed as the oils can change the nature of the fragrance.

Fragrance should be applied in the morning, at lunch, in late afternoon, and before bed. If your fragrance comes in a spray bottle, spray it 8 inches away from your body for proper dispersion. When you use your fingers to apply perfume from a bottle with a stopper, you can limit contamination of the fluid by not using the stopper as an applicator. Contaminants from your skin can stay on the stopper and be introduced into the perfume where they can incubate. Instead, use your fingers on the rim of the bottle.

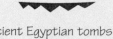

Ancient Egyptian tombs contained paintings of dashing playboys wearing fringed and pleated robes with tall braided and curled wigs upon which they balanced cones of fragrant ointments. The cones melted and oozed onto their wigs and garments, scenting them in the process.

Save your perfume for evening wear when you want a slightly stronger effect. However, if you have dry skin or find you have to reapply your scent too often, consider using a bit of perfume during the day. Apply your scent 10 to 15 minutes before a special occasion to give it time to settle down and mellow.

Do not spray scent directly on your clothes because perfume can stain fabrics and cling to them. If you want to scent your clothes, mist undergarments or your nightie, and put dusting powder in your shoes.

Store fragrance in a zip-seal bag when traveling.

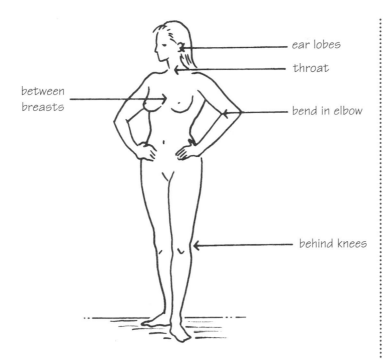

ear lobes

throat

between breasts

bend in elbow

behind knees

Apply fragrance at the pulse points shown several times a day.

CLIMATE, GEOGRAPHY, BODY CHEMISTRY, AND FRAGRANCE

When your skin perspires in hot weather, the natural oils and moisture amplify, and hold on to a perfume's fragrance. In the cold, your skin is drier, giving perfume nothing to hold on to so it evaporates quicker. Therefore heavier scents can be worn in the winter.

Perspiration and heat cause a fragrance to emanate and be more pronounced, so be sure to use the lightest form of your chosen scent when engaging in sports activities.

High altitudes decrease the long-lasting effects of fragrance so you will need to apply scent more often. Also, your fragrance will be perceived as being lighter, so you may want to try a stronger fragrance.

Other factors which will affect your body chemistry, and therefore your perfume, include medication, spicy or high fat foods, stress, and pregnancy.

SHOPPING FOR PERFUME

Build your fragrance wardrobe over time with different concentrations of scents such as eau de parfum, toilet water, and cologne. Remember, no matter how beautiful the bottle, it's what's inside that you must concentrate on. Considering the price of fine fragrances today, the time it takes to choose a perfect fragrance is a prudent investment. After all, your perfume may be the first impression that you give someone, so it should be memorable for all the right reasons.

In the store, spray fragrance onto a mouillette (perfume blotter paper) before applying it to your skin. Mouillettes are available at the perfume counter. Using them will help rule out scents you do not like before you apply them to your pulse points for long-term evaluation. Don't try more than three or four scents at one time as you will not be able to distinguish any more than that. Many stores have containers of coffee beans to sniff which refresh your ability to discern scents.

Take your time at the perfume counter. A fragrance needs at least fifteen to twenty minutes to fully develop and should not be judged until that amount of time has elapsed.

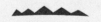

"Everyone has a personal scent circle which extends an arm's length from the body. No one should be aware of your fragrance unless he or she steps inside your circle."

—Annette Green
president of the Fragrance
Foundation, NYC

It's important to obtain a sample to take home with you so that you can try a fragrance several times, giving the perfume time to make an impression on you. Does it last a reasonable length of time? Do other people react favorably to the scent on you? Most importantly, does the fragrance make you feel wonderful and bring a smile to your lips? If not, do not buy it!

And finally, be aware that fragrance has a finite shelf life. Purchase only the amount you will use within 18 months.

CHAPTER 4

HOW TO CREATE YOUR OWN FRAGRANCES

There are lots of fragrance recipes for you to explore in the next two chapters. Let's start here with some basic definitions and how-tos.

THE DIFFERENCE BETWEEN PERFUME AND COLOGNE

The strength and longevity of a scent created to use on the body is ranked according to the concentration of essential or fragrance oils in an alcohol and distilled water base. Even though it's not listed, there is distilled water in every fragrance. In perfume, and eau de parfum, distilled water is present in the alcohol base. It is added as a separate ingredient in the lighter scents. In all cases, the presence of distilled water softens a fragrance and slows its evaporation rate.

Listed below, ranked from longest-lasting to lightest scent, are the gradations of fragrances for women. Please note that the longevity of any fragrance depends on the exact amount of essential or fragrance oils used, each person's individual body chemistry, and the circumstances under which the fragrance is worn. For example, a perfume worn by a person with dry skin living in a cold climate will not last as long as the same perfume worn by a person who has oily skin living in a warm climate.

Also, different families of perfume have vastly different staying powers once applied to the skin. A composition in the oriental family is far more tenacious than one in the citrus family, for example. Also remember that different notes in one blend have different longevities with top notes the most fleeting and base notes longest lasting. That's why it's important, when purchasing fragrance, to ask for a sample to take home. That way, you may apply the scent and live with it for a while before investing in a bottle.

THE VARIETIES OF SCENT

Perfume, or extrait, is the most concentrated form of fragrance and may contain up to 300 different elements in its blend with a 15 to 30 percent concentration of essential and fragrance oils in an alcohol base and a fragrance time of three to eight hours. Perfume is the longest lasting scented substance you can apply to your skin.

Eau de parfum is also long lasting, with an 8 to 15 percent concentration of essential and fragrance oils diluted in alcohol and distilled water base.

Eau de toilette is next in line, a lighter version of scent with a 4 to 8 percent concentration of essential and fragrance oils in an alcohol and distilled water base. It will last approximately four to six hours.

Eau de cologne is a less concentrated scented compound with a ratio of 2 to 5 percent of essential or fragrance oils in an alcohol and distilled water base. This form of fragrance was originally developed in Italy in the seventeenth century. However, it is named for the city of Cologne, Germany, because this is the place where it was first marketed successfully at the end of the eighteenth century. It is often used as an after-bath splash and will last for two to four hours.

Eau fraîche is the lightest scented substance, with a 1 to 3 percent concentration of perfume oils in alcohol and distilled water. Use a light splash of eau fraîche in hot weather or when engaging in sports. An old-fashioned term for eau fraîche is sweet water.

THE VARIETIES OF FRAGRANCE FOR MEN

Colognes are the most concentrated and longest-lasting forms of men's fragrance. They are meant to be used on the body rather than the face.

Aftershave comes in two forms. One features cooling, astringent qualities and is meant to heal small shaving nicks. The other is a newer variety, sometimes called balm, and it's designed to moisturize and smooth the skin. The scent in both varieties of aftershave is formulated to last only a short period of time.

Pre-shaves quicken the evaporation of moisture on the skin, stiffening the beard, and coating the skin so that an electric razor will perform more smoothly. They are very lightly scented. Some brands contain methanol, and all contain astringents which are helpful in preventing shaving rash.

Talcs are lightly scented powders which remove facial shine after shaving. They also help to prevent chafing and collar rub.

FRAGRANCE TIPS FOR MEN

A few drops of fragrance sprinkled on your handkerchief every morning will add a refreshing lift to your day.

Keep bars of soap in your sock drawer and sprinkle talc in your sneakers and gym bag.

BASIC EQUIPMENT FOR MAKING YOUR OWN FRAGRANCE

Making fragrances at home is not complicated but you do need to pay attention to the equipment you gather and the work area you set up for this process.

Work Area

Set up your work area so that it is convenient to hot water and with ample storage for your ingredients and equipment. I use a wall cabinet in my laundry room to store my oils and bases. This area is air-conditioned in the summer and well-ventilated at other times of the year so warmth and steam are not problems here. Any cool, dark room or a cool room with a cabinet will be a safe place to store your ingredients. If you have a room in your basement, this would be a good choice.

Be sure there is good ventilation in your work area because many of the essential and fragrance oils are quite aromatic in their undiluted state. Reserve the utensils you use for fragrance crafting for that purpose only.

Your work surface should be approximately 3 feet by 6 feet and covered with a plastic cloth. I like flannel-backed plastic cloths best because they stay in place well. Inexpensive folding tables or card tables are good choices for a work surface if they are sturdy.

Equipment

Measuring cups and spoons are necessities for fragrance crafting. Indulge yourself in a new glass measuring cup and a set of plastic measuring spoons. Be sure to clean the spoons with alcohol after each use so that traces of a previous scent won't contaminate the next.

A small glass pitcher or a beaker marked with measurements and with a pouring spout is very helpful for mixing.

A glass rod is the best implement to use for stirring because it does not become impregnated with scent as a wooden spoon will. Medical supply houses and laboratory suppliers are the best place to find these. Check your phone book or ask your local pharmacist for assistance finding a source.

Droppers are probably the most important piece of fragrance crafting equipment. And glass droppers are the best because they are the easiest to clean. Some pharmacies will sell you droppers at cost so you can have one for every oil you use. Simply tape the appropriate dropper to the essential oil bottle so it will be there the next time you compose a perfume. Over time, the rubber tops will become sticky and break down. When that happens, it's time to get a new dropper.

If you have only one dropper, wash it in hot, soapy water and rinse with isopropyl alcohol to avoid introducing a previously used oil into the next bottle. Be sure the dropper is

You will need a glass beaker, dropper, plastic measuring spoons, funnel, and a variety of dark glass bottles for making your own scents.

completely dry before using it again. A hair dryer can expedite this process.

A narrow funnel is useful for filling your bottles with your perfumes. Small perfume bottles with narrow openings require a tiny perfume funnel which is no more than an inch and a half high. Once when I misplaced my narrow funnel, I cut off the tip of a cone-shaped paper cup, which makes a great disposable funnel. Cut off just a tiny bit of the tip to fill perfume bottles. Cut off a bigger piece of the tip to funnel lotions, bath oils, or dusting powder. If a recipe calls for filtration, a paper coffee filter placed inside a plastic strainer will work. Always strain liquids until they are clear.

An electric coffee mill, set aside specifically for fragrance crafting, can be used to grind up whole spices and herbs.

Glass bottles, preferably blue, amber or green are best for storing your perfumes, sweet waters, and colognes. Bottles can be found in lots of places. (See the source guide on page 153.) Old perfume bottles, often found in garage sales, are perfect for fragrance crafting and you will be recycling at the same time. Be sure they are thoroughly washed in hot, soapy water, rinsed with isopropyl alcohol, and completely dried before using.

When looking for old perfume bottles to reuse, check them over carefully. Be sure there is no permanent residue inside. Also check to see if the stopper is a tight fit. If the bottle is corked, you will need to get a new cork at a craft store and seal the bottle with paraffin.

If the bottle you choose has a screw top, be sure the top has a liner, a small disc of material inside the cap to prevent the contents of the bottle from contacting the cap.

Lighter forms of fragrance, such as eau fraîche or splashes, can be stored in plastic bottles with tight-fitting tops, but stronger concentrations require glass containers.

Spray bottles are wonderful for splashes, rosewater, lavender flower, and orangeflower waters. Beauty supply stores and pharmacies often carry these bottles and they are quite inexpensive. Be sure to wash your new bottles before using.

CAUTION

Remember — do not use metal spoons, bowls, or funnels for your fragrance crafting. The metal will taint essential and fragrance oils.

CHOOSING THE RIGHT CONTAINER
FOR YOUR FRAGRANCES

Please be aware that you must choose the correct container for your fragrance. For example, containers made from HDPE will collapse if filled with perfume, perfume oil, eau de parfum, or cologne.

Container	Suitable for:
HDPE (high density polyethylene) frosted plastic	Bath gels only, lotions, eau fraîche, astringents, toners, bubble bath (do not use for oil-based products)
PVC or PET (polyvinyl chloride or polyethylene terephthalate) clear plastic	Bath oils, massage oils
Glass	Perfumes, perfume oils, eau de parfum, cologne

SEALING BOTTLES WITH PARAFFIN

Perfume bottles that are sealed with a cork should be sealed with paraffin also because corks breathe and allow your perfume to evaporate.

Purchase the paraffin used for canning at your local supermarket or hardware store. Place the paraffin in a coffee can in a pan filled with several inches of water. Turn the heat on low and allow the water to simmer and gently melt the paraffin.

Dip the cork-topped bottle into the melted paraffin, covering the whole surface of the cork thoroughly. Allow the wax to harden then repeat the process until the paraffin is thick enough to form a seal. If you like, you can melt a crayon in the paraffin to add color.

Do not, under any circumstances, leave the melting paraffin unattended, because it is flammable.

BASIC INSTRUCTIONS

While the ingredients in the recipes in chapters 5 and 6 are different, many of the processes of making fragrance are the same. Here are some general instructions that apply to every recipe you decide to try.

1. Containers should be clean, dry, and as sterile as possible. For best results, boil your bottles in hot water for ten minutes. Be sure to dry them thoroughly before using.
2. Always store your essential and fragrance oils and blends in a cool, dark place, as heat and light can alter the composition of your product. Do not store fragrances in the bathroom, as the heat and steam may have a damaging affect on them.
3. Changes in color or viscosity indicate a perfume is old and should be discarded. If you detect an "off" smell in any preparation, throw it out.
4. All fragrance blends should be tested for skin sensitivity. To test, apply a drop to the inside of your elbow. If there is no redness or reaction in 24 hours, the blend is safe to use.
5. Do not use essential or fragrance oils directly on your skin. Always dilute them with jojoba, sweet almond, or apricot kernel oil first.
6. Label everything that you make with the name and the date that you made it.
7. Never use metal containers or implements, as a chemical reaction may occur, altering your scent.
8. If glycerin is used in a recipe, blend it with the water in the recipe before adding the other ingredients in order to avoid bubbles.
9. Remember, all of the recipes in chapters 5 and 6 are fun ideas for gift giving or your own enjoyment. But if you are considering selling your preparations, the FDA requires you to use containers approved for cosmetic use.
10. If you want to put flowers in your blends for color and decoration, be sure they are chemical free.

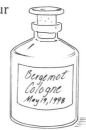

Be sure to label all your creations with the ingredients and the date of creation.

COMPOSING YOUR OWN FRAGRANCES

After you've tried a few of my recipes, I would encourage you to try your hand at composing your own fragrances. Here are some general blending guidelines for the different types of scented products you can make at home.

Ingredients Guidelines

◆ Amber adds warmth and sweetness to a blend.
◆ Bergamot adds a sunny, citrus scent to every blend.
◆ Carnation contains spicy eugenol which gives a clove-like fragrance.
◆ Frangipani is deliciously sweet and spicy.
◆ Frankincense adds a mellow, woody note to a blend.
◆ Heliotrope and violet enhance each other in a composition.
◆ Neroli adds a warm, dry note to a blend and balances the fragrance of rose.
◆ Oakmoss imparts a powdery, lichen scent to fragrance.
◆ Patchouli adds woodsy, earthy notes to a composition.
◆ Rosemary adds green, pine scents to a fragrance.
◆ Sandalwood imparts a warm, sensual note to a blend and is a delicious aroma all on its own.
◆ Tuberose is intensely sweet and heavy.
◆ Vanilla is a tenacious aroma that enhances, mellows, and sweetens any blend.
◆ Vetiver adds woodsy, musky notes to a fragrance.

Now let's move on to the fun of making your own fragrances.

CITRUS WARNING

Blends containing citrus oils, especially bergamot, should not be worn in the sun because they increase photosensitivity. However, you can purchase bergamot oil without bergaptene, the ingredient that causes this problem.

CHAPTER 5

RECIPES FOR PERFUMES, COLOGNES, AND SWEET WATERS

Now that you've determined your fragrance wardrobe, it's time to explore the scents you can make at home. Today the range of quality fragrance oils available to you is wonderful. However, you do get what you pay for, whether it's an essential or fragrance oil. Pure, undiluted essential oils can be tested by applying a few drops to a strip of blotter paper. If the oils are pure, they will evaporate leaving no oily residue. A quality synthetic fragrance oil will imitate a scent, so a gardenia oil should remind you of those creamy, velvety blossoms as you sniff the essence. When it comes to rose scents and blends, shop around for the one that pleases you the most.

When you buy ingredients for these recipes, bear in mind that the result depends on the quality of the oils you purchase. Be sure you are purchasing undiluted oils from a reputable dealer. There are several listed in the source guide on page 153.

A WORD ABOUT OILS

While it's always a good idea to use naturally derived, essential oils when creating a fragrance, some scents are either unavailable or prohibitively expensive for home use. For example, lily of the valley does not give up its fragrance so it's necessary to duplicate it in a laboratory, while rose or jasmine absolute costs thousands of dollars a pound. In the following recipes, I have specified which oils are essential oils. The other oils are synthetics.

When making perfumes, always add your fragrance or essential oils to the alcohol base first, then add the other ingredients. The alcohol allows the oils to blend with the other ingredients, especially the distilled water.

When buying fragrance or essential oils, be sure to read the label carefully. If the label says "oil of," the contents are essential oils. If the label says "_____" oil, the contents are fragrance oils. For example, oil of sandalwood is an essential oil. On the other hand, a bottle marked sandalwood oil is a fragrance oil.

While many of the ingredients in these recipes will be available in your local health food or grocery store, many of them are harder to find. For fragrance sources, see pages 153–155.

A WORD ABOUT VODKA AND WATER

The overall quality of each ingredient you use to make a fragrance affects the overall quality of the final product. For best results, I recommend you use a high-quality, 100-proof vodka as the base in the alcohol-based recipes because it has virtually no aroma of its own. Do not use rubbing alcohol as a substitute because it evaporates much too quickly and has a strong odor.

When a recipe calls for water, be sure to use bottled or distilled water. Tap water contains too many organisms and minerals which can destroy your fragrance.

BASIC PROPORTIONS

As you make any of these fragrance recipes, bear in mind that you can control the strength of the final product. This means if you like colognes better than perfumes, you can alter the recipe to fit your preference. The following list will tell you how to alter the amount of base in order to compose a fragrance to your specifications. All of these proportions assume you are using no more than 30–40 drops of fragrance or essential oils. Use less oil for heavier scents such as patchouli, sandalwood, rose, or vanilla. Use more for citrus scents. Remember you can always add more fragrance or essential oils if the scent, after having a chance to mellow, is not strong enough to suit you.

◆ **Perfume:** After selecting the essential or fragrance oils you want in your perfume, blend them and add ⅛ ounce of 100 proof vodka to the mixture.

◆ **Eau de Parfum:** After selecting the essential or fragrance oils you want in your eau de parfum, blend them and add ¼ ounce of 100 proof vodka to the mixture.

◆ **Eau de Toilette:** After selecting the essential or fragrance oils you want in your eau de toilette, blend them and add ½ ounce of 100 proof vodka to the mixture.

◆ **Sweet Waters:** In a four-ounce glass bottle, blend your oils then add one ounce of 100-proof vodka to the mixture. Fill the rest of the bottle with distilled water. Shake and allow to mellow for two weeks. Stir with a glass rod or gently swirl the contents every day.

◆ **Perfume Oil:** Jojoba is a liquid wax rather than an oil. It disappears into the skin after application and does not become rancid over time, which makes it a perfect base for perfume oils. To make perfume oil, follow the general instructions for making perfume but substitute jojoba in place of the vodka. Sweet almond or apricot kernel oil may also be used as a base but be aware that these oils have only a three to six month shelf life before they become rancid.

Keep in mind that you cannot substitute an oil base in a recipe that includes distilled water because the two will not mix.

Here at Gingham 'n' Spice, we've created fragrance crafting kits to help you begin your exploration of scent. The kits include rosewater, jojoba oil, glycerin, droppers, glass bottles, and six vials of fragrance. There is a kit for five of the fragrance families — floral, oriental, woodsy/spicy, green/chypre, and citrus. For ordering information, see page 153.

When you begin your fragrance crafting, it is all right to substitute fragrance oils for essential oils. The result will smell the same. However you will have a finer and longer lasting fragrance if you use essential oils. In any case, it is important to purchase only oils that you can smell while you're still in the store.

BASIC RECIPES

There are a few basic mixtures that appear in several of the recipes I've gathered for you. Some, like rosewater and orange-flower water, are wonderful to use all by themselves, either in your bath or as a refresher for your skin. Others, like tincture of benzoin, are for use only in a recipe.

ROSEWATER SPLASH

The finest rosewater is made from the prohibitively expensive rose otto or rose attar, extracted from the Bulgarian or damask rose. This is combined with distilled or deionized water to make a pure rosewater. Due to the high cost of rose oil, we are using a synthetic fragrance oil in this simple recipe. Use one cup in your bath, as an after-bath splash or in the recipes that follow. This splash makes a wonderful toner after cleansing your skin to hydrate and normalize its acid balance. Use within one month after aging one to two weeks.

2 cups distilled water
½ cup red rose petals (chemical free)
20 drops rose fragrance oil

1. Gently pull the rose petals from the flower head. When measuring this ingredient, do not pack the petals down.
2. Pour the distilled water into a glass or plastic bottle.
3. Add rose petals and rose oil and stir.
4. Seal the bottle and store in a cool, dark place for 1–2 weeks. Stir the contents with a glass rod or gently swirl the ingredients every few days.

ROSEWATER

If you are going to make a recipe that calls for rosewater, I would recommend you purchase rosewater made with rose attar. This top quality rosewater is alcohol-free and gentle enough to use as a freshener on sensitive skin or on the skin around the eyes. I include this recipe so you can make your own rosewater, but be aware that it contains alcohol and will not be as gentle or hydrating as high-quality, commercial rosewater. The alcohol is necessary for its preservative and sterilization properties.

2 cups distilled water
4 tablespoons vodka
½ cup fresh, chemical-free rose petals (choose fragrant varieties such as damask or others mentioned in the fragrant flower chart on page 149)

1. Combine the ingredients in a sterilized glass bottle.
2. Stir gently with a glass rod or swirl the contents.
3. Store in a cool, dry place for a week.
4. Strain out the rose petals using a strainer lined with muslin or a paper coffee filter.
5. Bottle and enjoy. If you use pink roses rather than red, you may wish to add one drop of red food coloring to add a pink cast to your rosewater.

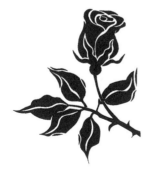

Try sprinkling uncolored rosewater, orange-flower water or any of the other sweet water recipes in this chapter onto linens as you iron them for a delicate bit of fragrance.

ORANGEFLOWER WATER

This sweet water is wonderful both by itself and in conjunction with other oils.

16 ounces distilled water
2 ounces vodka
25 drops essential oil of bergamot
14 drops essential oil of sweet orange

1. Measure and pour the distilled water and vodka into a sterilized glass bottle.
2. Add the bergamot and sweet orange oils and stir.
3. Seal the bottle and store in a cool, dark place for 1–2 weeks. Stir with a glass rod or gently swirl the contents every few days.
4. Shake well before using.

TINCTURE OF BENZOIN

Floral waters such as rosewater, orangeflower water, Florida water (see page 79), and lavender water will last longer if ⅛ ounce tincture of benzoin is added to each cup of liquid. This tincture will make the floral water turn milky. Shake these fragrant waters well before using.

1 part powdered benzoin
6 parts vodka

1. Mix the ingredients in a sterile glass bottle.
2. Shake the mixture periodically until the powdered material is completely dissolved. This should happen within a day. Tincture is also available premixed.

ORRIS ROOT TINCTURE

Orris root tincture is added to perfume as a fixative.

1 part powdered orris
root
20 parts vodka

1. Combine the orris root with the vodka and mix thoroughly.
2. Strain through muslin or a paper coffee filter.
3. Store in a sealed, glass bottle. Shake well before using.

RECIPES WITH A HISTORY

You can enjoy the history of fragrance by making the following classic recipes. They're just as wonderful today as they were centuries ago.

FLORIDA WATER

This is an American version of the original Eau de Cologne, introduced in this country in 1808.

2 cups distilled water
¼ cup vodka
6 drops essential oil of
lavender
2 drops essential oil of
clove bud
8 drops essential oil of
bergamot

1. Pour the water and vodka into a sterilized glass container.
2. Add the lavender, clove bud, and bergamot oils, stirring well.
3. Seal the bottle and store in the refrigerator for two weeks so that the scents will be well blended.
4. Use within two months if you keep this mixture refrigerated, two weeks if not.

HUNGARY WATER

This is the first alcohol-based perfume in history, developed for Queen Elizabeth of Hungary in 1370.

1 lemon or orange
1 cup orangeflower water
1 teaspoon glycerin
1 cup vodka
½ teaspoon essential oil of lemon
2 teaspoons essential oil of bergamot
⅛ teaspoon essential oil of rosemary
2 tablespoons fresh peppermint leaf, cut into small pieces (use 1 tablespoon if peppermint is dried)

1. Sterilize a glass container.

2. Cut from your orange or lemon a continuous peel that's long enough to fit top to bottom in your container. A handy kitchen tool called a zester is great at making one continuous peel. Also be aware that it is the skin of the fruit and not the white pulp which contains the oil you want for this recipe.

3. Blend the orangeflower water and glycerin.

4. Add the vodka to the orangeflower water and glycerin combination, then add the peppermint leaf and the essential oils.

5. Cap the glass container tightly and place it in a cool, dark place for 2–4 weeks (the longer the better).

6. Decant your Hungary Water into a perfume bottle, using a coffee filter or muslin to strain out the peppermint leaf and citrus peel.

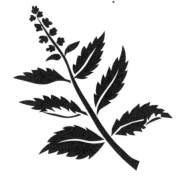

EAU DE COLOGNE

This recipe is as close to the original Eau de Cologne as you can make at home, a delightful fragrance.

½ cup vodka
12 drops essential oil of bergamot
18 drops essential oil of lemon
20 drops essential oil of petitgrain
4 drops essential oil of neroli
4 drops essential oil of rosemary
2 tablespoons orange-flower water

1. Sterilize a glass container.
2. Measure the vodka into the glass.
3. Add the bergamot, lemon, petitgrain, neroli, and rosemary oils and the vodka. Cap tightly.
4. Let the vodka and oil mixture sit for two days.
5. After two days, add the orangeflower water.
6. Let the mixture sit for two more days before straining through cheesecloth or a coffee filter and rebottling.
7. Use within twelve months.

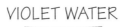

VIOLET WATER

Parma violets are still cultivated and their essences distilled at the San Giovanni Parma monastery in Evangelista, Italy. Violet fragrances were favored by Marie-Antoinette and by the Victorians.

The quantity of vodka in this recipe will preserve this fragrant combination indefinitely.

8 tablespoons vodka
4 tablespoons distilled water
10 drops violet fragrance oil

1. Sterilize a glass container.
2. Pour the vodka and distilled water into the glass.
3. Add the violet oil.
4. Store in a cool, dark place and let the mixture age for a week or two.

CARMELITE WATER

In 1379, nuns from the Abbaye St. Juste made Carmelite water for Charles V of France. Angelica and other herbal oils went into the compound. This is a delightful sweet water.

1 lemon
4 ounces vodka
3 tablespoons chopped lemon balm leaves
3 tablespoons chopped angelica root
½ teaspoon coriander seeds
1 nutmeg
1 3-inch cinnamon stick
1 tablespoon whole cloves

1. Sterilize a glass container.
2. Peel the lemon with a zester.
3. Pour vodka into the glass.
4. Add the lemon balm leaves and angelica root to the vodka.
5. Grate the nutmeg and add to the vodka mixture.
6. Add the lemon peel, cinnamon stick, and cloves. Stir.
7. Cap tightly, store in a cool, dark place, and let sit for 3 to 4 weeks, shaking the bottle every day.
8. Strain the Carmelite water through a paper coffee filter or muslin as you decant it into your perfume bottle.
9. Use within twelve months.

LAVENDER WATER

Twelfth-century Abbess Hildegard of Bingen on the Rhine is thought to have created the first lavender water. The word lavender comes from the Latin *lavare* (to wash) and has long been linked to cleanliness.

Since you are using actual oils and not lavender blossoms in this recipe, your sweet water will be fragrant upon completion. Aging will mellow the results. My lavender water is still fragrant and perfect after a year.

2 cups of distilled water
2 ounces vodka
10–20 drops essential oil of lavender

1. Sterilize a glass container.
2. Pour the distilled water and vodka into the glass.
3. Add the lavender oil and stir.

RECIPES FOR THE FLORAL FAMILY OF FRAGRANCES

This is by far the largest family of scents and can even include flowers from your garden. For information about growing fragrant flowers for your garden, see page 152.

FLOWER WATER

In the summer, I keep this mixture in the refrigerator to freshen my skin after being overheated. It is quite soothing.

½ cup rosewater
¼ cup orangeflower water

1. Sterilize a glass container.
2. Combine the rosewater and orangeflower water in the glass. You can use this recipe right away.
3. Add ¼ cup of witch hazel to the above blend and you will have a lovely mild astringent.

ROSE COLOGNE

The glycerin and tincture of benzoin in this recipe act as preservatives, so this fragrant mixture will last a long time. Since glycerin is also a moisturizer, this is good for your skin too.

If you use an essential oil of rose, this will be a finer blend. However, essential rose oil is expensive so I suggest you test synthetic rose oils to find one you like in order to contain costs.

2 cups distilled water
2 tablespoons glycerin
1 cup vodka
¾ teaspoon rose
    fragrance oil
¾ teaspoon essential oil
    of rose geranium
1 tablespoon tincture of
    benzoin

1. Sterilize a glass container.
2. Combine the water and glycerin, stirring well to prevent bubbles from forming. Add the vodka. Shake well.
3. Add the rose and geranium oils, then the tincture of benzoin. The mixture will turn milky when the tincture is added. Shake well.
4. Cap tightly and store in a cool, dark place for 1 to 2 weeks. Stir with a glass rod or swirl the contents gently every few days.
5. Shake well before using.

WOODROSE PERFUME

The blend of rose and sandalwood in this recipe is heavenly.

¼ cup rosewater
1 cup vodka
2 tablespoons rose
   fragrance oil
1 teaspoon essential oil
   of sandalwood

1. Sterilize a glass container.
2. Pour the rosewater and vodka into the glass.
3. Add the rose and sandalwood oils, then shake the container vigorously.
4. Store in a cool, dark place for 3 to 4 weeks, shaking daily.

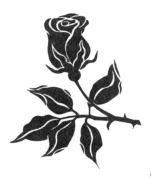

SOUTHERN BELLE

Patchouli deepens and mellows the luscious florals in this blend. East Indian patchouli is the highest quality oil.

4 drops lilac fragrance oil
8 drops rose fragrance oil
8 drops jasmine
   fragrance oil
12 drops gardenia
   fragrance oil
5 drops essential oil of
   East Indian patchouli

For perfume: Fill a sterilized ½-ounce glass bottle with ¾ teaspoon vodka and add the scented oils in the order given.

For perfume oil: Fill a sterilized ½-ounce glass bottle with ¾ teaspoon jojoba oil, apricot kernel oil, or sweet almond oil. Add the scented oils in the order given.

ROSE JAR

This an old-fashioned rose scent.

8 drops essential oil of verbena

12 drops rose fragrance oil

6 drops essential oil of sandalwood

6 drops essential oil of East Indian patchouli

For perfume: Fill a sterilized ½-ounce glass bottle with ¾ teaspoon vodka and add the scented oils in the order given.

For perfume oil: Fill a sterilized ½-ounce glass bottle with ¾ teaspoon jojoba oil, apricot kernel oil, or sweet almond oil. Add the scented oils in the order given.

LOVE'S PROMISE

Spicy carnation lights up the floral and fruity notes in this blend, which is warmed all over by musk.

2 drops peach fragrance oil

10 drops rose fragrance oil

6 drops carnation fragrance oil

8 drops lily of the valley fragrance oil

6 drops musk fragrance oil

For perfume: Fill a sterilized ½-ounce glass bottle with ¾ teaspoon vodka and add the scented oils in the order given.

For perfume oil: Fill a sterilized ½-ounce glass bottle with ¾ teaspoon jojoba oil, apricot kernel oil, or sweet almond oil. Add the scented oils in the order given.

SILK SHANTUNG

Sweet jasmine and mimosa are topped with neroli (also known as orange blossom) and fixed with frankincense.

8 drops essential oil of neroli

12 drops mimosa fragrance oil

6 drops jasmine fragrance oil

6 drops essential oil of frankincense

For perfume: Fill a sterilized ½-ounce glass bottle with ¾ teaspoon vodka and add the scented oils in the order given.

For perfume oil: Fill a sterilized ½-ounce glass bottle with ¾ teaspoon jojoba oil, apricot kernel oil, or sweet almond oil. Add the scented oils in the order given.

MEMORIES

This blend crosses the floral line into the oriental family to make it a floriental. Heady tuberose and gardenia form the middle notes of this recipe, with the citrus scent of bergamot as a top note and a warm sandalwood base.

6 drops essential oil of bergamot

16 drops tuberose fragrance oil

4 drops essential oil of ylang-ylang

6 drops gardenia fragrance oil

8 drops essential oil of sandalwood

For perfume: Fill a sterilized ½-ounce glass bottle with ¾ teaspoon vodka and add the scented oils in the order given.

For perfume oil: Fill a sterilized ½-ounce glass bottle with ¾ teaspoon jojoba oil, apricot kernel oil, or sweet almond oil. Add the scented oils in the order given.

RECIPES FOR THE FRUITY FAMILY OF FRAGRANCES

These perfumes have a clean, light fragrance with just a few citrus notes.

PEARWOOD

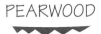

Juicy pear notes meld with the citrus scents of petitgrain and lemon verbena, then are warmed by a luscious sandalwood and vanilla base. This is a long-lasting scent.

12 drops pear fragrance oil

4 drops essential oil of lemon verbena

2 drops essential oil of petitgrain

8 drops vanilla fragrance oil

4 drops essential oil of sandalwood

For perfume: Fill a sterilized ½-ounce glass bottle with ¾ teaspoon vodka and add the scented oils in the order given.

For perfume oil: Fill a sterilized ½-ounce glass bottle with ¾ teaspoon jojoba oil, apricot kernel oil, or sweet almond oil. Add the scented oils in the order given.

FRUIT 'N' SPICE

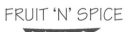

The peach and pear notes are brightened by nutmeg and cinnamon then blend with the base note of vanilla.

12 drops pear fragrance oil

4 drops peach fragrance oil

2 drops essential oil of cinnamon

3 drops essential oil of nutmeg

8 drops vanilla fragrance oil

For perfume: Fill a sterilized ½-ounce glass bottle with ¾ teaspoon vodka and add the scented oils in the order given.

For perfume oil: Fill a sterilized ½-ounce glass bottle with ¾ teaspoon jojoba oil, apricot kernel oil, or sweet almond oil. Add the scented oils in the order given.

RECIPES FOR THE GREEN FAMILY OF FRAGRANCES

The green family of fragrances are for those of you who love the outdoors and the scent of new-mown hay.

VIOLET PERFUME

1½ cups vodka
¼ cup distilled water
¾ teaspoon violet
   fragrance oil
¾ teaspoon rose
   fragrance oil
4 drops essential oil of
   bergamot
1 tablespoon orrisroot
   tincture

1. In a sterilized glass bottle, mix the vodka and water.
2. Add the oils in the order specified in the recipe.
3. Add the orrisroot tincture and stir well. The tincture will make your blend cloudy.
4. Shake well before using.

BREATH OF SPRING

Green top notes of hyacinth predominate, resting on lily of the valley, and cyclamen middle notes on an oakmoss base.

12 drops hyacinth
   fragrance oil
8 drops lily of the valley
   fragrance oil
6 drops cyclamen
   fragrance oil
4 drops essential oil of
   oakmoss

For perfume: Fill a sterilized ½-ounce glass bottle with ¾ teaspoon vodka and add the scented oils in the order given.
For perfume oil: Fill a sterilized ½-ounce glass bottle with ¾ teaspoon jojoba oil, apricot kernel oil, or sweet almond oil. Add the scented oils in the order given.

EMERALD HERBS

Top notes of lavender and rosemary are highlighted by the green notes of violet and oakmoss's chypre base note.

4 drops essential oil of rosemary

12 drops essential oil of lavender

4 drops violet fragrance oil

8 drops essential oil of oakmoss

For perfume: Fill a sterilized ½-ounce glass bottle with ¾ teaspoon vodka and add the scented oils in the order given.

For perfume oil: Fill a sterilized ½-ounce glass bottle with ¾ teaspoon jojoba oil, apricot kernel oil, or sweet almond oil. Add the scented oils in the order given.

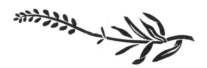

APRIL SHOWERS

In this blend, hyacinths and violets herald spring's arrival with the earthy scents of lavender, cedarwood, and patchouli.

6 drops essential oil of lavender

12 drops violet fragrance oil

6 drops hyacinth fragrance oil

4 drops essential oil of East Indian patchouli

4 drops essential oil of cedarwood

For perfume: Fill a sterilized ½-ounce glass bottle with ¾ teaspoon vodka and add the scented oils in the order given.

For perfume oil: Fill a sterilized ½-ounce glass bottle with ¾ teaspoon jojoba oil, apricot kernel oil, or sweet almond oil. Add the scented oils in the order given.

RECIPES FOR THE SPICY FAMILY OF FRAGRANCES

These are pungent scent recipes, full of nutmeg, ginger, cloves, and cinnamon.

SPICED ROSEWATER

This is a piquant version of the rosewater recipe on page 77.

1 cup rosewater
1 tablespoon whole cloves
1 nutmeg
2 cinnamon sticks
4 drops essential oil of
lavender

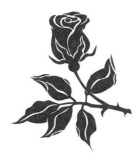

1. Sterilize a glass container.
2. Measure out and pour the rosewater into the glass.
3. Crush the cloves, nutmeg, and cinnamon sticks and add to the rosewater. A hammer is the best tool to use to crush the nutmeg.
4. Add the lavender oil. Cap tightly.
5. Store in a cool, dark place for 2 weeks.
6. Strain through a paper coffee filter or muslin and decant into your perfume bottle.
7. Use within 2 weeks.

SECRETS

The lavender and rose in this blend are heightened by spicy notes of cinnamon and allspice, then mellowed by base notes of sandalwood.

4 drops essential oil of
allspice
2 drops essential oil of
cinnamon
10 drops essential oil of
lavender
10 drops rose fragrance oil
4 drops essential oil of
sandalwood

For perfume: Fill a sterilized ½-ounce glass bottle with ¾ teaspoon vodka and add the scented oils in the order given.
For perfume oil: Fill a sterilized ½-ounce glass bottle with ¾ teaspoon jojoba oil, apricot kernel oil, or sweet almond oil. Add the scented oils in the order given.

COLOGNES

ISLAND SPICE EAU DE TOILETTE

An amber glass bottle tied with jute and a few bay leaves makes this recipe a nice gift for a man or a woman.

2 cups vodka
1 nutmeg, broken
3 cinnamon sticks
2 tablespoons coriander seeds
1 orange, zest only
2 bay leaves
1 tablespoon cloves, whole

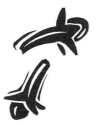

1. Sterilize a glass container.
2. Pour the vodka into the glass.
3. Crush the cinnamon sticks and coriander seeds and add to the vodka.
4. Remove the orange zest in spirals. If your bay leaves are fresh, use them whole. If they are dried, break them up before adding to your blend so they will fit into your glass container. Add the orange zest, bay leaves, nutmeg, and whole cloves to the vodka mixture.
5. Cap the bottle tightly and let sit in a warm, dark place, such as a kitchen cupboard, for 2 weeks.
6. Strain through a paper coffee filter or muslin and pour into a glass bottle. Add the orange peel to the bottle, and a cinnamon stick if you wish.

DELIGHT

Nutmeg and lavender complement each other in this blend. These top notes rest on a heart of rose and a base of vanilla and sandalwood.

4 drops essential oil of nutmeg
6 drops essential oil of lavender
6 drops rose fragrance oil
4 drops essential oil of sandalwood
12 drops vanilla oil

For perfume: Fill a sterilized ½-ounce glass bottle with ¾ teaspoon vodka and add the scented oils in the order given.
For perfume oil: Fill a sterilized ½-ounce glass bottle with ¾ teaspoon jojoba oil, apricot kernel oil, or sweet almond oil. Add the scented oils in the order given.

AUTUMN LEAVES

This is vanilla and spice with a sweet orange heart.

2 drops essential oil of allspice
4 drops essential oil of cinnamon
8 drops essential oil of sweet orange
16 drops vanilla fragrance oil

For perfume: Fill a sterilized ½-ounce glass bottle with ¾ teaspoon vodka and add the scented oils in the order given.
For perfume oil: Fill a sterilized ½-ounce glass bottle with ¾ teaspoon jojoba oil, apricot kernel oil, or sweet almond oil. Add the scented oils in the order given.

RECIPES FOR THE ORIENTAL FAMILY OF FRAGRANCES

The French use the word amber to describe the full-bodied, woodsy aroma of the oriental family of fragrance. This heavy-scented family does not lend itself to the lighter forms of fragrance such as eau fraîche or sweet waters.

FRENCH VANILLA AND TEA ROSE PERFUME

I use vanilla oil in many of my recipes as a base note. I find it to be a wonderful addition that softens and rounds out a blend enhancing the other ingredients in the process. This recipe straddles the line between floral and oriental families.

⅓ cup vodka
1 tablespoon rosewater
1 cup chemical-free rose petals
2 vanilla beans, whole
10 drops vanilla fragrance oil
10 drops essential oil of petitgrain
5 drops rose fragrance oil

1. Sterilize a glass container.
2. Combine the vodka and rosewater in the glass.
3. Add the vanilla beans and the oils.
4. Cap tightly and store in a cool, dark place for two to three weeks.
5. Strain and add a rosebud or two if you wish. A drop of red vegetable food coloring may be added for a hint of pink. If red rose petals are used this may not be necessary.

CRÈME DE VANILLE COLOGNE

Find a pretty bottle to display this cologne in. Crème de Vanille is one of my favorites. This is a great recipe for teens too.

¼ cup vodka
¼ teaspoon glycerin
1 vanilla bean
4 drops heliotrope
  fragrance oil
1 orange or lemon
A few dried or fresh rosebuds (optional)

1. Sterilize a glass container.
2. Combine the vodka and glycerin in the glass. Shake vigorously.
3. Split the vanilla bean lengthwise and add to the vodka mixture.
4. Add the heliotrope oil.
5. Use a zester to peel a 3-inch strip of orange or lemon peel, taking care to take only the zest, not the white pulp. Add to the vodka mixture. Shake.
6. Store in a cool, dark place and age for at least 1 week. Stir with a glass rod or gently swirl contents after a few days.
7. Decant into a decorative jar. If desired, you can add rosebuds to this recipe after it has aged. Strip the leaves and stems from your chemical-free rosebuds, leaving the petals and calyx behind. Add them to the mixture for color and decoration.

TUSSIE MUSSIE

Vanilla and sandalwood add the oriental touch to this bouquet of florals.

2 drops essential oil of
  ylang-ylang
8 drops gardenia
  fragrance oil
4 drops jasmine fragrance
  oil
8 drops vanilla fragrance
  oil
6 drops essential oil of
  sandalwood

For perfume: Fill a sterilized ½-ounce glass bottle with ¾ teaspoon vodka and add the scented oils in the order given.
For perfume oil: Fill a sterilized ½-ounce glass bottle with ¾ teaspoon jojoba oil, apricot kernel oil, or sweet almond oil. Add the scented oils in the order given.

MYSTERY

Jasmine and gardenia blend with bois de rose and amber notes for a decidedly oriental blend.

12 drops gardenia fragrance oil
6 drops jasmine fragrance oil
6 drops essential oil of bois de rose
6 drops amber fragrance oil

For perfume: Fill a sterilized ½-ounce glass bottle with ¾ teaspoon vodka and add the scented oils in the order given.

For perfume oil: Fill a sterilized ½-ounce glass bottle with ¾ teaspoon jojoba oil, apricot kernel oil, or sweet almond oil. Add the scented oils in the order given.

WEDDING BLISS

This recipe combines stephanotis (a favorite of brides) with delightful honeysuckle and the vanilla-almond notes of heliotrope on a vanilla base. This a great recipe for teens too.

10 drops essential oil of heliotrope
8 drops honeysuckle fragrance oil
8 drops stephanotis fragrance oil
6 drops vanilla fragrance oil

For perfume: Fill a sterilized ½-ounce glass bottle with ¾ teaspoon vodka and add the scented oils in the order given.

For perfume oil: Fill a sterilized ½-ounce glass bottle with ¾ teaspoon jojoba oil, apricot kernel oil, or sweet almond oil. Add the scented oils in the order given.

WOOD ROSE

Rose and honeysuckle are freshened with top notes of bergamot and warmed with sandalwood.

6 drops essential oil of bergamot

10 drops rose fragrance oil

8 drops honeysuckle fragrance oil

8 drops essential oil of sandalwood

For perfume: Fill a sterilized ½-ounce glass bottle with ¾ teaspoon vodka and add the scented oils in the order given.

For perfume oil: Fill a sterilized ½-ounce glass bottle with ¾ teaspoon jojoba oil, apricot kernel oil, or sweet almond oil. Add the scented oils in the order given.

IVY ROSE

A lovely combination of rose and violet lightly spiced with clove bud and the herbal green notes of rose geranium. The balsam imparts a woody note.

2 drops essential oil of clove bud

4 drops essential oil of rose geranium

8 drops rose fragrance oil

10 drops violet fragrance oil

8 drops essential oil of balsam

For perfume: Fill a sterilized ½-ounce glass bottle with ¾ teaspoon vodka and add the scented oils in the order given.

For perfume oil: Fill a sterilized ½-ounce glass bottle with ¾ teaspoon jojoba oil, apricot kernel oil, or sweet almond oil. Add the scented oils in the order given.

SPICE ISLAND

*S*picy notes of cinnamon, mace, and carnation blend with lavender and rest on a warm base of vanilla.

10 drops essential oil of
   lavender
8 drops vanilla fragrance
   oil
4 drops essential oil of
   cinnamon
4 drops carnation
   fragrance oil
2 drops essential oil of
   mace

For perfume: Fill a sterilized ½-ounce glass bottle with ¾ teaspoon vodka and add the scented oils in the order given.

For perfume oil: Fill a sterilized ½-ounce glass bottle with ¾ teaspoon jojoba oil, apricot kernel oil, or sweet almond oil. Add the scented oils in the order given.

RECIPES FOR THE CITRUS FAMILY OF FRAGRANCES

The tang of lemon, the sweet, heady aroma of fresh orange, and the clean scent of lime are all in this fragrance family.

CITRUS GROVE

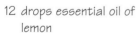

*L*emon and orange oils are fixed in a base of clary sage.

12 drops essential oil of
   lemon
7 drops essential oil of
   mandarin
2 drops essential oil of
   neroli
7 drops essential oil of
   tangerine
4 drops essential oil of
   clary sage

For perfume: Fill a sterilized ½-ounce glass bottle with ¾ teaspoon vodka and add the scented oils in the order given.

For perfume oil: Fill a sterilized ½-ounce glass bottle with ¾ teaspoon jojoba oil, apricot kernel oil, or sweet almond oil. Add the scented oils in the order given.

VERBENA SPLASH

This recipe produces a clean, fresh, lemony splash and is appropriate for both men and women.

1 cup lemon verbena leaves
½ cup vodka
8 drops essential oil of lemon verbena
2 orange peel strips, approximately 3"–4" long
1 cup distilled water

1. Sterilize a glass container.
2. If your verbena leaves are fresh, bruise them before adding. If they are dried, crush them lightly and put into container.
3. Add the vodka and verbena oil and cover tightly.
4. Infuse for 2 weeks in a cool, dark place, stirring with a glass rod or gently swirling the contents once a week.
5. Add orange peel for the last 2 days of the infusion period.
6. Strain through a paper coffee filter or muslin cloth.
7. Add distilled water and shake thoroughly.
8. Use within two weeks if not refrigerated, within four weeks if it is refrigerated.

NECTAR

This fresh and lively fragrance is appropriate for both men and women.

6 drops essential oil of sweet orange
8 drops essential oil of lemon
8 drops essential oil of tangerine
6 drops essential oil of frankincense
4 drops essential oil of neroli

For perfume: Fill a sterilized ½-ounce glass bottle with ¾ teaspoon vodka and add the scented oils in the order given.
For perfume oil: Fill a sterilized ½-ounce glass bottle with ¾ teaspoon jojoba oil, apricot kernel oil, or sweet almond oil. Add the scented oils in the order given.

SUMMERTIME

Orange and tangerine sweeten this wonderful warm weather fragrance. This is a good recipe for teens too.

8 drops essential oil of tangerine
6 drops essential oil of sweet orange
10 drops essential oil of heliotrope
8 drops vanilla fragrance oil

For perfume: Fill a sterilized ½-ounce glass bottle with ¾ teaspoon vodka and add the scented oils in the order given.

For perfume oil: Fill a sterilized ½-ounce glass bottle with ¾ teaspoon jojoba oil, apricot kernel oil, or sweet almond oil. Add the scented oils in the order given.

MELODY

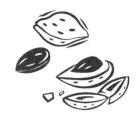

The scent of amaretto and blooming gardenia mix with the dry note of neroli for this intriguing fragrance. Teens love this recipe too.

4 drops essential oil of neroli
10 drops gardenia fragrance oil
6 drops almond fragrance oil
12 drops vanilla fragrance oil

For perfume: Fill a sterilized ½-ounce glass bottle with ¾ teaspoon vodka and add the scented oils in the order given.

For perfume oil: Fill a sterilized ½-ounce glass bottle with ¾ teaspoon jojoba oil, apricot kernel oil, or sweet almond oil. Add the scented oils in the order given.

NOTE ON THE MODERN FAMILY OF FRAGRANCES

Recipes for the modern family of fragrances are all based on aldehydes, which are not readily available to the home fragrance crafter, so no recipes are included here.

RECIPES FOR THE CHYPRE FAMILY OF FRAGRANCES

These warm, alluring scents are perfect for evening wear. Their distinct aroma is based on woodsy notes such as oakmoss, lavender, patchouli, and vetivert.

CYPRESS ISLE

This heavenly scent is laced with the earthy tones of cedarwood.

6 drops essential oil of bergamot
6 drops peach fragrance oil
8 drops jasmine fragrance oil
6 drops essential oil of oakmoss
4 drops essential oil of cedarmoss

For perfume: Fill a sterilized ½-ounce glass bottle with ¾ teaspoon vodka and add the scented oils in the order given.
For perfume oil: Fill a sterilized ½-ounce glass bottle with ¾ teaspoon jojoba oil, apricot kernel oil, or sweet almond oil. Add the scented oils in the order given.

MOSSY GLEN

The heady aroma of ylang-ylang weaves through this perfume.

8 drops essential oil of lemon
6 drops essential oil of ylang ylang
4 drops rose fragrance oil
8 drops essential oil of oakmoss
4 drops essential oil of vetiver

For perfume: Fill a sterilized ½-ounce glass bottle with ¾ teaspoon vodka and add the scented oils in the order given.
For perfume oil: Fill a sterilized ½-ounce glass bottle with ¾ teaspoon jojoba oil, apricot kernel oil, or sweet almond oil. Add the scented oils in the order given.

EARTH FLOWER

The earthy aroma of patchouli blended with the spicy scent of carnations makes this chypre composition outstanding.

8 drops essential oil of bergamot

3 drops essential oil of clary sage

6 drops lily of the valley fragrance oil

4 drops carnation fragrance oil

4 drops essential oil of East Indian patchouli

6 drops essential oil of vetiver

For perfume: Fill a sterilized ½-ounce glass bottle with ¾ teaspoon vodka and add the scented oils in the order given.

For perfume oil: Fill a sterilized ½-ounce glass bottle with ¾ teaspoon jojoba oil, apricot kernel oil, or sweet almond oil. Add the scented oils in the order given.

ROCK GARDEN

Mossy notes from oakmoss blend with the dry, citrus notes of verbena in this chypre blend.

8 drops essential oil of lemon verbena

12 drops lily of the valley fragrance oil

6 drops rose fragrance oil

4 drops essential oil of oakmoss

For perfume: Fill a sterilized ½-ounce glass bottle with ¾ teaspoon vodka and add the scented oils in the order given.

For perfume oil: Fill a sterilized ½-ounce glass bottle with ¾ teaspoon jojoba oil, apricot kernel oil, or sweet almond oil. Add the scented oils in the order given.

MOONSHADOW

Victorian violet notes are laced with nutmeg and herbaceous lavender.

12 drops violet fragrance oil

8 drops essential oil of lavender

6 drops essential oil of oakmoss

4 drops essential oil of nutmeg

For perfume: Fill a sterilized ½-ounce glass bottle with ¾ teaspoon vodka and add the scented oils in the order given.

For perfume oil: Fill a sterilized ½-ounce glass bottle with ¾ teaspoon jojoba oil, apricot kernel oil, or sweet almond oil. Add the scented oils in the order given.

RECIPES FOR MEN

Men's fragrances rely on the earthy qualities of ingredients such as lavender, the sparkling scents of citrus, and bases such as bay leaf, sandalwood, and vetiver.

NOTE ON THE OCEANIC FAMILY OF FRAGRANCES

The recipes for the oceanic family of fragrances are so complex that they are not appropriate for home fragrance crafting.

HERBAL AFTERSHAVE

The presence of glycerin in this recipe makes this aftershave good for the skin.

1 cup vodka
2 teaspoons glycerin
½ teaspoon essential oil of lemon
10 drops essential oil of clove bud
½ teaspoon essential oil of rosemary
½ teaspoon essential oil of lavender
2 drops tincture of benzoin

Combine all ingredients and seal in a glass bottle. Shake before using.

BAY RUM AFTERSHAVE

You can use either whole fresh or broken dried bay leaves for this recipe.

4 ounces vodka
2 bay leaves
2 tablespoons Jamaican rum
1 cinnamon stick, whole
½ teaspoon allspice, whole
Zest from 1 orange
10 drops essential oil of clove bud
50 drops essential oil of bay

Combine all ingredients and cap tightly in a glass bottle. Age for 2 weeks, then strain and discard solids. Add fresh or dried bay leaves if you wish, especially if you are giving this as a gift.

KEY LIME COLOGNE

The prevailing lime notes in this blend combine with orange for this wonderful aftershave splash.

1 cup vodka
Zest from 2 limes
18 drops essential oil of lime
12 drops essential oil of petitgrain
6 drops essential oil of bergamot
6 drops essential oil of bay
1 cup orangeflower water
1 teaspoon tincture of benzoin

Add lime zest to the vodka and infuse for one week.

Add remaining ingredients. Cap tightly and age for 4 weeks. Strain through a paper coffee filter or muslin cloth and enjoy.

BAYWOOD

A top note of clove bud and the spicy notes of bayberry and juniper are rounded out with a base of vanilla and long lasting sandalwood.

2 drops essential oil of clove bud
8 drops essential oil of juniper
6 drops bayberry fragrance oil
10 drops vanilla fragrance oil
6 drops essential oil of cedarwood

For perfume: Fill a sterilized ½-ounce glass bottle with ¾ teaspoon vodka and add the scented oils in the order given.

For perfume oil: Fill a sterilized ½-ounce glass bottle with ¾ teaspoon jojoba oil, apricot kernel oil, or sweet almond oil. Add the scented oils in the order given.

For a lighter scent: Blend your oils in a four-ounce glass bottle then add 2 tablespoons of 100-proof vodka to the mixture. Fill the rest of the bottle with distilled water. Shake and allow to mellow for 2 weeks. Unlike perfume or perfume oil, this lighter version of fragrance needs time for the essential and fragrance oils to permeate the vodka and water base. Stir with a glass rod or gently swirl the contents every day.

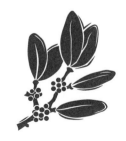

PROVENCE

The ingredients in this blend make it a traditional men's scent.

4 drops essential oil of ginger
14 drops essential oil of lavender
4 drops essential oil of cedarwood
6 drops essential oil of sandalwood
2 drops essential oil of vetiver

For perfume: Fill a sterilized ½-ounce glass bottle with ¾ teaspoon vodka and add the scented oils in the order given.

For perfume oil: Fill a sterilized ½-ounce glass bottle with ¾ teaspoon jojoba oil, apricot kernel oil, or sweet almond oil. Add the scented oils in the order given.

For a lighter scent: Blend your oils in a four-ounce glass bottle then add 2 tablespoons of 100-proof vodka to the mixture. Fill the rest of the bottle with distilled water. Shake and allow to mellow for 2 weeks. Stir with a glass rod or gently swirl the contents every day.

HARBOR LIGHTS

Herbal spicy notes are complemented by bergamot's orange scent.

10 drops essential oil of bergamot
6 drops essential oil of allspice
4 drops essential oil of lavender
12 drops essential oil of bay leaf

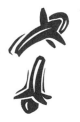

For perfume: Fill a sterilized ½-ounce glass bottle with ¾ teaspoon vodka and add the scented oils in the order given above.

For perfume oil: Fill a sterilized ½-ounce glass bottle with ¾ teaspoon jojoba oil, apricot kernel oil, or sweet almond oil. Add the scented oils in the order given.

For a lighter scent: Blend your oils in a four-ounce glass bottle then add 2 tablespoons of 100-proof vodka to the mixture. Fill the rest of the bottle with distilled water. Shake and allow to mellow for 2 weeks. Stir with a glass rod or gently swirl the contents every day.

FIRESIDE

This woody composition is a great fragrance for men. It has herbal notes and an enriching base of frankincense and myrrh.

6 drops essential oil of juniper

6 drops essential oil of pine

4 drops essential oil of myrrh

6 drops essential oil of cedarwood

8 drops essential oil of sandalwood

4 drops essential oil of frankincense

For perfume: Fill a sterilized ½-ounce glass bottle with ¾ teaspoon vodka and add the scented oils in the order given.

For perfume oil: Fill a sterilized ½-ounce glass bottle with ¾ teaspoon jojoba oil, apricot kernel oil, or sweet almond oil. Add the scented oils in the order given.

For a lighter scent: Blend your oils in a four-ounce glass bottle then add 2 table-spoons of 100-proof vodka to the mixture. Fill the rest of the bottle with distilled water. Shake and allow to mellow for 2 weeks. Stir with a glass rod or gently swirl the contents every day.

FOREST

A wonderful fragrance for men. Forest notes prevail in this woodsy blend.

6 drops essential oil of pine needle

12 drops essential oil of balsam

6 drops essential oil of cedarwood

6 drops essential oil of patchouli

For perfume: Fill a sterilized ½-ounce glass bottle with ¾ teaspoon vodka and add the scented oils in the order given.

For perfume oil: Fill a sterilized ½-ounce glass bottle with ¾ teaspoon jojoba oil, apricot kernel oil, or sweet almond oil. Add the scented oils in the order given.

For a lighter scent: Blend your oils in a four-ounce glass bottle then add 2 table-spoons of 100-proof vodka to the mixture. Fill the rest of the bottle with distilled water. Shake and allow to mellow for 2 weeks. Stir with a glass rod or gently swirl the contents every day.

RECIPES FOR TEENS

Young women between the ages of twelve and twenty enjoy lighter fragrances. These recipes are sure to be a hit with them.

HONEYBEE SWEET WATER

Honey is the oldest known humectant and still one of the best for keeping the skin moisturized. This is a very refreshing splash or toner with a fresh, natural scent.

2 tablespoons honey
2 teaspoons fresh lemon juice, strained
4 tablespoons vodka
2 tablespoons rosewater

1. Sterilize a glass container.
2. Stir the honey and lemon juice together until combined.
3. Add the vodka and rosewater. Stir well with a glass rod and the mixture will be ready to use.
4. Use within 2 months.

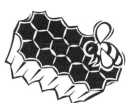

BLUSHING ROSE

This is a sweet and rosy blend with the zip of lemon verbena.

8 drops essential oil of lemon verbena
10 drops essential oil of ylang-ylang
8 drops rose fragrance oil
6 drops amber fragrance oil

For perfume: Fill a sterilized ½-ounce glass bottle with ¾ teaspoon vodka and add the scented oils in the order given.
For perfume oil: Fill a sterilized ½-ounce glass bottle with ¾ teaspoon jojoba oil, apricot kernel oil, or sweet almond oil. Add the scented oils in the order given.

APPLE DUMPLING

Apple and raspberry top notes are blended with spices then warmed by vanilla. Yum!

12 drops apple fragrance oil
6 drops raspberry fragrance oil
2 drops essential oil of cinnamon or clove bud
2 drops essential oil of nutmeg
6 drops vanilla fragrance oil

For perfume: Fill a sterilized ½-ounce glass bottle with ¾ teaspoon vodka and add the scented oils in the order given.

For perfume oil: Fill a sterilized ½-ounce glass bottle with ¾ teaspoon jojoba oil, apricot kernel oil, or sweet almond oil. Add the scented oils in the order given.

PROM NIGHT

Fragrant gardenia, spicy carnation, a garden of roses, and lavender combine with a vanilla base for a special fragrance.

4 drops carnation fragrance oil
6 drops essential oil of lavender
4 drops rose fragrance oil
10 drops gardenia fragrance oil
8 drops vanilla fragrance oil

For perfume: Fill a sterilized ½-ounce glass bottle with ¾ teaspoon vodka and add the scented oils in the order given.

For perfume oil: Fill a sterilized ½-ounce glass bottle with ¾ teaspoon jojoba oil, apricot kernel oil, or sweet almond oil. Add the scented oils in the order given.

PARADISE

This fruity oriental blend is electrified by ginger then mellowed by a vanilla base note.

4 drops essential oil of ginger
10 drops peach fragrance oil
8 drops coconut fragrance oil
8 drops vanilla fragrance oil

For perfume: Fill a sterilized ½-ounce glass bottle with ¾ teaspoon vodka and add the scented oils in the order given.

For perfume oil: Fill a sterilized ½-ounce glass bottle with ¾ teaspoon jojoba oil, apricot kernel oil, or sweet almond oil. Add the scented oils in the order given.

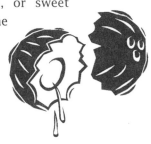

SWEET NOTHINGS

An oriental base of amber, sandalwood, and vanilla support the lovely floral notes of heliotrope and ylang-ylang.

8 drops essential oil of heliotrope
4 drops essential oil of ylang-ylang
8 drops vanilla fragrance oil
8 drops amber fragrance oil
2 drops essential oil of sandalwood

For perfume: Fill a sterilized ½-ounce glass bottle with ¾ teaspoon vodka and add the scented oils in the order given.

For perfume oil: Fill a sterilized ½-ounce glass bottle with ¾ teaspoon jojoba oil, apricot kernel oil, or sweet almond oil. Add the scented oils in the order given.

SERENITY

The fragrant notes of ylang-ylang are sparked with citrus notes and warmed by base notes of vanilla.

3 drops essential oil of lemon

8 drops essential oil of bergamot

3 drops essential oil of sweet orange

6 drops essential oil of ylang ylang

8 drops vanilla fragrance oil

For perfume: Fill a sterilized ½-ounce glass bottle with ¾ teaspoon vodka and add the scented oils in the order given.

For perfume oil: Fill a sterilized ½-ounce glass bottle with ¾ teaspoon jojoba oil, apricot kernel oil, or sweet almond oil. Add the scented oils in the order given.

RECIPES FOR UNISEX FRAGRANCES

Some fragrance recipes are just right for both genders and all ages. The citrus notes keep these blends fresh and sparkling.

SUNNY CITRUS COLOGNE

This cologne is refreshing and appropriate for men or women.

2 cups vodka

Zest from 1 orange

Zest from 1 lemon

1 cup of orangeflower water

12 drops essential oil of sweet orange

12 drops essential oil of lemon verbena

6 drops essential oil of bergamot

1. Sterilize a glass container.

2. Pour vodka into the container.

3. Add the orange and lemon zests.

4. Cap tightly and store in a cool, dark place to infuse for 1 week.

5. Strain and add remaining ingredients. Shake well.

6. Return container to cool, dark place and age mixture for 2 to 4 more weeks.

GERANIUM TOILET WATER

This is a fresh scent with decidedly green notes.

1 cup vodka
1 cup distilled water
1 cup scented geranium
  leaves (rose, lemon-
  rose, lime, or nutmeg)
½ cup lavender flowers
  (the tiny buds)
4 drops essential oil of
  rose geranium

1. Sterilize a glass container.
2. Combine the vodka and distilled water in the container.
3. If you are using smaller geranium leaves, such as those on the nutmeg geranium, use the whole leaf. If the leaves you have are larger, you can roll them into a tube shape and insert them whole into the container. Or you may bruise larger leaves, tear them into pieces, and put them in the glass container.
4. If you grow your own lavender, strip the blossoms from the stem with your fingers. Add them to the mixture.
5. Add the geranium oil and cap tightly.
6. Store in a cool, dark place for 2 weeks, shaking the container every few days.
7. Strain through a paper coffee filter or muslin and store in an appropriate bottle.
8. Use within 2 months.

FRENCH SORBET

Lemon, lime, and the orange notes of bergamot are held together with a frankincense base.

12 drops essential oil of
  bergamot
10 drops essential oil of
  verbena
8 drops essential oil of
  lime
6 drops essential oil of
  frankincense

For perfume: Fill a sterilized ½-ounce glass bottle with ¾ teaspoon vodka and add the scented oils in the order given.
For perfume oil: Fill a sterilized ½-ounce glass bottle with ¾ teaspoon jojoba oil, apricot kernel oil, or sweet almond oil. Add the scented oils in the order given.

BERGAMOT COLOGNE

Try refrigerating this fresh eau de cologne during the summer months.

½ cup vodka
Zest from 1 orange
1 teaspoon whole cloves
1 teaspoon whole allspice
6 drops essential oil of
    bergamot

1. Sterilize a glass container.

2. Pour vodka into container.

3. Add the orange peel, whole cloves, all-spice, and bergamot oil. Shake well.

4. Cap tightly and store in a cool, dry place for 1 to 2 weeks or until the scent is the strength you prefer.

5. Strain through a paper coffee filter or muslin and bottle.

6. Use within 12 months.

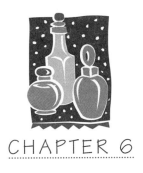

CHAPTER 6

MORE FORMS OF FRAGRANCE: BATH SALTS, INCENSE, AND MORE

Why stop at perfume and cologne when there are bath salts, dusting powder, solid and cream perfumes, incense, and potpourri? Fragrance is a wonderful part of life, and I always think the more, the better.

BATH SALTS

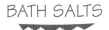

This is one of the easiest forms of fragrance to create at home. And at the end of a long day, what can be better than a soak in a hot tub of scented water?

If you're giving this as a gift, include a large scallop shell as a scoop.

2 cups Epsom salts
¾ cup powdered milk
½ cup borax
1½ teaspoons fragrance oil, essential oil, or fragrance blend
1–2 drops food coloring (optional)

If you decided to add the food coloring to your bath salts, mix the dry ingredients and food coloring in a non-metallic bowl with a wooden spoon that you reserve for fragrance crafting only. Or you may measure all the dry ingredients and the food coloring into a locking plastic bag and mix thoroughly. Once they are mixed, add the fragrance oil and mix again.

Water softener salt may be substituted for Epsom salts but be sure not to use anything larger than a medium crystal because it won't dissolve properly.

Use ⅓ to ½ cup of bath salts in the tub.

DUSTING POWDER

Extend the longevity of a perfume or cologne with a complementary dusting powder of the same fragrance. If you're giving this as a gift, add a swansdown puff.

2 cups arrowroot or cornstarch
½ cup baking soda
½–1 teaspoon fragrance, essential, or blended oil

Blend all ingredients well. Pass through a seive to remove any lumps. Store in a glass shaker or a recycled talcum powder dispenser.

CALMING FLOWER BATH OIL

Turkey red oil is the only oil that will disperse in water rather than float on top. If you're going to give this as a gift, add a loofah sponge or a fancy scrubber of net or foam.

1 cup turkey red oil (sulfonated castor oil)
30–40 drops fragrance, essential, or blended oil
or
10 drops rose fragrance oil
10 drops essential oil of lavender
10 drops essential oil of sandalwood
10 drops vanilla fragrance oil

Combine the turkey red oil and your choice of scent. Shake well. Use 2 tablespoons per bath.

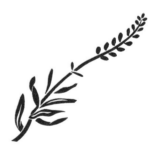

SILKY HAND LOTION

The rosewater in this recipe will help hydrate your skin every time you use this lotion.

½ cup rosewater
½ cup glycerin

Blend the ingredients well and store in a sealed bottle.

SOLID OR CREAM PERFUMES

Solid and cream perfumes can be carried in unspillable versions. Moisturizing and pleasant to use, plus, they're easy to whip up in 10 or 15 minutes.

2 tablespoons grated
beeswax
2 tablespoons sweet
almond oil
1–2 teaspoons essential or
fragrance oils

1. Melt beeswax in an enamel or glass pan over boiling water. Add sweet almond oil; combine. Be patient with this step; it's important to blend them completely.

2. Allow the mixture to cool slightly before adding the oils of your choice (suggestions follow).

3. Fill clean, dry glass jars with the solid perfume.

Hint: After step 1, you may add 1 tablespoon of distilled water if you want a firmer result.

COMBINATIONS OF SCENTS

Lovenotes
1 teaspoon essential oil of lavender
1/2 teaspoon essential oil of bergamot
1/8 teaspoon essential oil of allspice

Romantic Moments
1/2 teaspoon vanilla oil
1/2 teaspoon gardenia oil

Orchard Fruits
1/2 teaspoon apple oil
1/2 teaspoon pear oil
1/2 teaspoon peach oil

Valley Green
1 teaspoon hyacinth oil
1/2 teaspoon chypre or oakmoss oil
1/2 teaspoon violet oil

Orient Express
1 teaspoon essential oil of
frankincense
1/2 teaspoon essential oil of myrrh
1/4 teaspoon essential oil of
sandalwood

Sunny Citrus

½ teaspoon essential oil of sweet orange
½ teaspoon essential oil of lemon
½ teaspoon essential oil of bergamot

Woodlands

½ teaspoon essential oil of cedarwood
½ teaspoon essential oil of sandalwood
½ teaspoon essential oil of bay

ENVIRONMENTAL FRAGRANCE

All of our wonderful scented products, from perfume to bath oil, from aftershave to sweet waters, began with the environmental fragrances of the ancient world. The following recipes will give you ideas for adding lovely fragrances to your whole world.

Incense and Burning Perfumes

Incense probably originated in the sweet woods and resins thrown on ancient fires. Ancient Egyptians burned several substances in their worship of the sun god Ra — resin as he rose, myrrh when he was overhead, and a mixture of 16 ingredients as he set in the west. There are references to the burning of incense in carvings and fragments of paintings from Babylon, recipes for its production in the Bible, and references to it in writings by the Greek physician Galen.

Incense, sometimes called burning perfume, can be an oil sprinkled on a heat source. It can be a combination of dried materials to be heated in a brazier on a wood stove or thrown directly on a fire. Or incense can be formed into cones or sticks to be burned.

BASIC SPICE MIX

This mixture is the base for many of the incense recipes that follow. It is not meant to be burned by itself.

1 tablespoon each of the following ground spices: cinnamon, cloves, mace, and allspice

Measure and mix together.

VICTORIAN ROSE BURNING PERFUME

This fragrance was favored by Victorian ladies.

¼ cup damask roses,
   crushed
¾ teaspoon frankincense,
   powdered
1 tablespoon Basic Spice
   Mix (see page 114)
¾ teaspoon orrisroot,
   powdered
½ cup rosewater
6 drops rose fragrance oil
6 drops musk fragrance oil

Combine roses, frankincense, and Spice Mix. Mix orrisroot with rosewater, and add to spice mixture. Add rose and musk oils and mix well.

BURNING DRY INCENSE

Put a few spoonfuls of any of these dried incense recipes in a small metal dish such as a tart tin. Place the dish in a 200–250°F oven with the door ajar, or on the back of a wood stove. A delicate aroma will waft throughout the room.

WOODS 'N' SPICE INCENSE

This is a relaxing fragrance with a delicious scent.

1 ounce frankincense
   tears
1 ounce myrrh pebbles
1 ounce vetiver, cut into
   1" pieces
1 tablespoon Basic Spice
   Mix (see page 114)
¾ teaspoon essential oil of
   lavender
½ teaspoon essential oil of
   sandalwood or cedarwood

Combine ingredients. You may also add lavender buds, rose petals, cloves, sandalwood chips, or cinnamon chips.

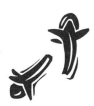

SWEET MYSTERY INCENSE

This is a spicy citrus blend laced with lavender and rose.

½ cup powdered orrisroot
½ cup frankincense tears
1 tablespoon Basic Spice Mix (see page 114)
¾ teaspoon essential oil of sweet orange
¾ teaspoon essential oil of clove bud
¾ teaspoon essential oil of lemon verbena
¾ teaspoon rose fragrance oil
½ cup lavender buds
¼ cup whole cloves
¼ cup cinnamon sticks, broken

Mix orrisroot, frankincense tears, spice mix and oils. Blend thoroughly and add to remaining ingredients.

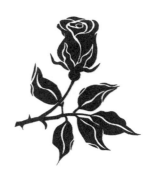

Scented Joss Sticks

Search your local stores for unscented joss sticks or "punks." Soak in your favorite scented oils. Let dry and burn as incense sticks. Try soaking some in citronella oil, dry them, and then place in a flowerpot filled with sand. Insects will stay away from your next picnic or barbecue.

Potpourri

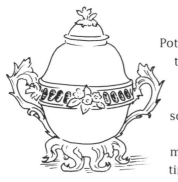

Potpourris were found in most rooms in Colonial times. The word potpourri comes from the French verb *pourrir* which means to rot and since these mixtures were kept in a pot from which they scented a room, potpourri became rotted pot.

Potpourris can be made moist or dry and their main ingredient is traditionally roses. In Colonial times, the most popular form of potpourri was a moist mixture, consisting of wilted flowers, mainly roses, layered with salt, bay leaves, brown sugar, and brandy. After the crock was filled, a weight was placed on top of the mixture and it was stirred periodically. The finished potpourri was kept in a rose jar, and when a room was cleaned, the jar was opened to perfume the air because ventilation was considered unsafe.

Manor houses had stillrooms where the lady of the house put together her own special recipes for potpourris and linen closet sachets. Stillroom recipe books became treasured heirlooms.

COLONIAL ROSE POTPOURRI

This is a typical moist potpourri based on historical recipes. The rose petals and lavender should be partially dried before you begin making this potpourri.

10 cups rose petals (a fragrant variety such as damask)
2 cups lavender buds
½ cup orrisroot, powdered
8 bay leaves
2 cups sea salt or kosher coarse salt
½ cup allspice, crushed
½ cup crushed cinnamon sticks
½ cup cloves, crushed
½ cup brown sugar
½ cup brandy

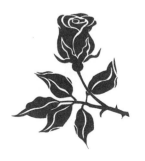

1. Mix the rose petals, lavender buds, and orrisroot powder together.
2. In a separate bowl, combine the bay leaves, salt, allspice, cinnamon, cloves and brown sugar.
3. In a large crock, layer the flowers with the spice mixture until all are used up.
4. Pour the brandy slowly over the top and put a weight such as a brick on top of the petals and cover the crock.
5. Stir every few days for 4–6 weeks until the scent pleases you. If desired, add 1 or 2 teaspoons of rose fragrance oil and additional spices.
6. Keep covered except when you remove the lid to scent the room.
7. Each year, add ½ cup of brandy and stir to renew the fragrance. It should last for many years.

COUNTRY KITCHEN SPICE POTPOURRI

This potpourri has a warm "welcome home" aroma that's pleasant any time of year.

1 tablespoon aniseed
1 tablespoon allspice
6 nutmegs
6 cinnamon sticks, coarsely broken
1 teaspoon powdered ginger
¼ cup whole cloves
1 teaspoon ground cinnamon
1–2 vanilla beans, cut into 1" pieces
1 cup coarse salt such as kosher salt

1. Crush aniseed and allspice in a mortar and pestle.
2. Use a hammer to crack the nutmeg and cinnamon sticks.
3. Mix all of the ingredients together and fill a lidded container of your choice. Old Mason jars work well.
4. Open whenever you want to freshen the air.

COTTAGE ROSE POTPOURRI

In order to dry the flowers in this potpourri, place them on paper towels in a warm, dry place such as the kitchen, attic, or garage until cornflake crisp.

Cellulose, made from crushed, dried corncobs, makes a wonderful base for potpourri. It is available from many of the sources listed in the source guide on page 153. Although orris root from the florentine iris is a fine fixative, I recommend you use cellulose because some people are very allergic to orris.

1 cup cellulose
⅛ ounce rose fragrance oil
30 drops essential oil of lemon verbena
20 drops essential oil of sandalwood
4 cups rose petals and buds
2 cups lemon verbena
2 cups patchouli
2 cups lavender buds

1. Mix the oils with the cellulose and store for two days in a jar with a tight-fitting lid.
2. Combine the dry potpourri ingredients with the oil/cellulose mixture and store for two to four weeks to allow the potpourri to age and develop. Do not use metal utensils, containers, or bowls as a reaction with the oils can adversely affect your final fragrance.

SPICED APPLE CIDER POTPOURRI

This potpourri is a medley of fall and winter aromas to remind us of home.

1 cup cellulose
⅛ ounce spiced apple fragrance oil
20 drops essential oil of cinnamon
4 cups dried red roses
2 cups dried apple slices
1 cup cinnamon sticks, broken
1 cup orange peel, dried
1 cup mulling spices (see page 120) or 1 cup whole cloves
2 cups pine cones (small, such as hemlock)

1. Mix the oils with the cellulose and store for two days in a jar with a tight fitting lid.

2. Combine the dry potpourri ingredients with the oil/cellulose mixture and store for 2 to 4 weeks to allow the potpourri to age and develop. Do not use metal utensils, containers, or bowls as a reaction with the oils can adversely affect your final fragrance.

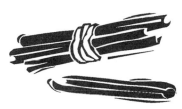

PRESERVING APPLE SLICES

There are ways to preserve apple slices to eat later and ways to preserve apple slices for use in potpourri, dried wreaths, or in floral baskets. To make these (inedible) dried apple slices, cut an unpeeled fruit into slices ¼ inch thick. Delicious apples should be sliced from top to bottom so their heart shapes will be preserved. Slice other types of apples crosswise.

Place the slices in a mixture of two cups lemon juice and one tablespoon salt for three minutes. Then arrange the slices in a single layer on a rack in a 150°F oven for six hours. The door of the oven should be left open and the slices turned if their edges begin to curl. When the apple slices are dry, they should feel leathery and be pliable.

MULLING SPICES

Mulling spices are used in warm apple cider or wine. They impart a spicy flavor to the brew. You can make your own or check in specialty shops for this tasty combination of spices.

¼ cup cinnamon sticks, broken into small pieces
¼ cup whole allspice
¼ cup whole cloves
¼ cup dried orange peel
¼ cup whole star anise
¼ cup nutmegs, broken (use a hammer)

Combine all ingredients and store in a sealed container.

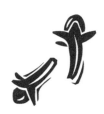

DEEP IN THE FOREST POTPOURRI

This woodsy blend is deepened by patchouli oil and a touch of spice. Cedar tips come from the last 3 to 4 inches of cedar branches.

4 cups cedar tips
4 cups pine cones, hemlock or spruce
2 cups berries — juniper or rosehips
1 cup cinnamon sticks, broken into 1" pieces
1 cup cellulose
¾ teaspoon essential oil of pine, balsam, or spruce
20 drops essential oil of patchouli
20 drops vanilla fragrance oil

Combine all ingredients and store in a sealed container.

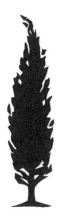

Sachets and Sweet Bags

"Sweet bag" is an old name for a small sachet bag made with a loop of ribbon in the top. Sweet bags are made to hang in closets, on the backs of chairs, or on doorknobs.

Sachets are scent-filled bags without a ribbon to hang them. Use sachets in linen closets, drawers, under seat cushions, in suitcases, and as shoe fresheners. Tie small sachets to coat hangers or hang them on a hook in the bathroom where the steam will intensify the scent.

Muslin, silk, or lightweight cotton fabric work best for sachets. Since I do not sew, I prefer collecting old handkerchiefs at flea markets for my sachets. I simply put a cup of my favorite sachet recipe in the center of the handkerchief, draw up the corners, and tie it with a pretty ribbon.

LEMON VERBENA SACHET

This recipe fills the room with the refreshing scent of lemon.

1 cup lemon verbena, dried and crushed fine

1 cup lemon balm, dried and crushed fine

1 cup rosemary, dried and crushed fine

1 teaspoon ground cloves

1 teaspoon ground mace or nutmeg

4 drops essential oil of sweet orange

1. Mix all ingredients together.
2. Keep the sachet mixture in a closed container for two weeks in order for scents to blend.
3. Fill small and medium-sized bags with the sachet mixture.

ROSE GERANIUM SACHET

My husband Bill grows all different kinds of scented geraniums which makes this blend a family affair. Any type of scented geranium will work in this recipe. Lime and apricot or nutmeg and cinnamon are especially nice.

This blend is very fresh smelling and belongs in the green fragrance family.

15 drops rose fragrance oil or essential oil of rose geranium

2 tablespoons sandalwood powder

2 cups rose geranium leaves, dried and crushed fine

2 cups rose petals, dried and crushed fine

1. Stir the oil into the sandalwood powder.

2. Combine with remaining ingredients and store in a covered container until you are ready to fill your sachets.

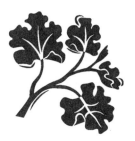

"SCENT YOUR OWN" SACHET POWDER

8 ounces arrowroot or cornstarch powder

2 ounces baking soda

1 ounce orrisroot powder

1 tablespoon salt

25 drops of essential oil, your choice

1. Combine the arrowroot or cornstarch, baking soda, and orris root. Allow to dry uncovered overnight.

2. Add the essential or fragrance oil to the salt.

3. Blend the salt mixture with the cornstarch mixture.

4. Fill and seal a glass container with the sachet powder and allow to mellow for 1 to 2 weeks.

STILLROOM SPICY SACHET

This recipe is based on recipes developed in Colonial stillrooms, the places where women created the healing potions used by their families.

You can gather your own balsam or pine needles for this recipe. Lavender buds should be stripped from the plant and allowed to dry on paper towels or a screen in a warm, dry place.

2 cups lavender buds
1 cup oakmoss, cut and sifted
1 cup dried balsam or pine needles
2 tablespoons ground cloves
2 tablespoons ground cinnamon
1 tablespoon ground ginger or nutmeg

1. Mix all ingredients together.
2. Keep the sachet mixture in a closed container for two weeks in order for scents to blend.
3. Fill small and medium sized bags with the sachet mixture.

Pomanders

King Baldwin of Constantinople introduced pomanders to Europe in 1174 when he presented one to Emperor Frederick Barbarossa during the crusades. Fashioned from gold and silver and decorated with jewels, pomanders were originally filled with musk but were later filled with ambergris. In fact, the word pomander comes from the French phrase *pomme d'ambre* (apple of amber). Some pomanders resembled a sectioned fruit with each part containing a different scent.

Prior to the sixteenth century, pomanders were attached to rosaries made of dried rosebuds or beads fashioned from aromatic substances. During the sixteenth century, they were attached to clothing in such a way that they would override the unsavory smells of the medieval streets.

The pomander that most of us are familiar with — an orange studded with cloves — was introduced to Europe by the Arabs. It was used to ward off pestilence and germs. Other variations of this pomander were hollowed-out apples and oranges containing mixtures of ambergris, frankincense, myrrh, and spices.

SPICE BATH FOR POMANDERS

Since spices should not be kept for more than a year, this is a great way to use up your out-of-date kitchen spices. You can hang this pomander in a closet to repel moths and impart its lovely fragrance or display it in a simple bowl with sprigs of greenery for a spicy centerpiece.

1 small orange
2 ounces whole cloves (per fruit)
1 tablespoon powdered orrisroot
1 tablespoon cinnamon, ground
1 tablespoon ground cloves, nutmeg or ginger, or a mixture of all three

1. Use a knitting needle, toothpick or awl to make small holes in the orange for the cloves.

2. Cover the whole fruit with cloves.

3. If you wish to hang the pomander, put a skewer or knitting needle through the center of the orange before rolling it in the spice bath.

4. Mix the spices you have chosen with the orrisroot and the cinnamon. Sprinkle in a shallow dish.

5. Roll the clove-studded orange in the spice bath mixture every few days until the fruit is dry.

6. If you want to hang your pomander, use a crochet hook to thread a ribbon or cord through the hole in the orange. Tie the ends of the ribbon or cord into a bow or knot to keep the ball from slipping off.

CASSOLETTES AND VINAIGRETTES

Cassolettes are small boxes with pierced lids containing aromatics which are meant to be inhaled. They were originally made from ivory, silver or gold. Cassolettes could be necklaces of hollow beads, or special rings with tops that opened to be filled with aromatic gums and perfumed powders, or silver earrings with hollow orbs containing bits of fabric that were soaked in perfume.

Vinaigrettes came into use after the pomander and also originated in France. Metalsmiths crafted small boxes of gold or silver with pierced lids and gilded interiors. These exquisite little boxes contained sponges soaked in vinegars distilled from acetate of copper and scented with rose, lavender, mint, rosemary, camphor, or other herbs. Flat and rectangular in shape, vinaigrettes were popular in Europe from the eighteenth century through the nineteenth century.

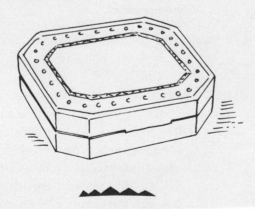

Other Ways to Use Fragrance in Your Home

Fragrance can enhance your environment in many ways. For example, many people dislike the smell of camphor. If so, the following recipe is for you.

MOTH AND INSECT REPELLENT

1 cup cedar chips
1 cup rosemary
1 tablespoon ground cloves
1 cup southernwood
1 tablespoon ground mace
1 cup lavender buds
¼ cup whole cloves
1 cup patchouli
1 cup peppermint leaves

Mix all ingredients together. Place a few spoonfuls of this mixture in a muslin or linen bag or a paper envelope. Place the bag or envelope in the linen closet or drawers where woolens are stored. It is important that the woolens be cleaned before storage.

LINEN CUPBOARD FRESHENER

This fragrance will permeate your linens, leaving them smelling fresh and clean.

2 tablespoons essential oil of lavender
3 cups coarse salt
12 cups lavender buds
1 cup coriander, crushed
6 nutmegs, cracked
½ cup allspice berries, crushed

1. Add the oils to the salt.
2. Layer lavender, spices, and salt mixture in a stone crock or glass jar until they are all used up. Weigh the mixture down with a heavy object such as a brick.
3. Stir after ten days and fill pint canning jars with the mixture. Glue a circle of fabric to the ring portion of the jar's lid, remove the circular insert, and screw the lid on the jar. Place jars in your linen closets or anywhere you want clothes to smell fresh.

SCENTED FURNITURE POLISH

8 ounces unrefined
  beeswax
2 ounces pure soap
  flakes or castile soap
1 pint turpentine
1 pint distilled water
30 drops essential oil of
  lavender, sandalwood,
  cedarwood, rosemary,
  or lemon verbena

1. Using a cheese grater, grate the beeswax and, if using castile soap, the soap.

2. In a double boiler over low heat, dissolve the beeswax in the turpentine. Remove the mixture from the heat as soon as the beeswax is dissolved.

3. In a separate pan, heat the water and dissolve the soap in it.

4. Pour the beeswax and soap mixtures into a bowl. Stir until cool.

5. Add the oil of your choice and stir the mixture.

6. Pour into an airtight container such as a canning jar with a lid. Let the polish harden overnight before sealing the jar. Then feed your furniture with this creamy, aromatic polish.

SCENTED INK

2 ounces ink
80 drops essential or
  fragrance oil
1 teaspoon vodka

Combine the vodka and oil. Slowly add this combination to your ink. Be sure to shake well before using.

If you're using essential oils, I suggest frankincense, patchouli, rose geranium, or lavender. If a synthetic oil is your preference, try rose, violet, carnation, or hyacinth.

Candles and Soap

There are any number of scented candles on the market today. There are also some incredible soaps and they make a wonderful tuck-in for a scented gift.

If you would like to try making your own scented candles or soap, you will find very complete directions in *The Candlemaker's Companion* by Betty Oppenheimer and Susan Cavitch's *The Natural Soap Book* from Storey.

Other Ways to Add Fragrance to Your Life

◆ Shelf paper or leftover wallpaper can be scented with your favorite perfume and used to line drawers. Simply spray your scent on the back side of the paper, let it dry, and line your drawers.

◆ Stationary can bear your signature scent. Simply sprinkle sachet powder in your stationery box under the paper and envelopes. If you use a fountain pen or a pen with a nib, you can scent your ink with a few drops of essential or fragrance oil too.

◆ Put cottonballs scented with a few drops of essential or fragrance oil in your dresser drawers.

◆ The next time you wrap a package, add a spritz of scent or a dot of perfumed oil to the ribbon.

◆ Put a few drops of perfume oil on a cool light bulb. When the light is turned on, the heat diffuses the oil. A note of caution here: never put oil on a hot bulb because it may break.

◆ Spray the towels in your bathroom with your favorite eau de toilette.

◆ A tissue or paper towel sprayed with scent and dropped into your wastebasket keeps it smelling pleasantly fresh.

CHAPTER 7

PACKAGING YOUR FRAGRANCES

I love to package my fragrances in pretty ribbons, paper, and decorated boxes. Here are some of my favorite ideas to get you started.

DECORATING BOXES

Many craft stores carry papier mâché boxes in a variety of shapes and sizes that are strong enough to hold bath salts, dusting powder, potpourri, or a bottle of perfume. Dusting powder or bath salts can be put into a plastic bag and then placed inside a papier mâché box. There are many ways to decorate these boxes.

You can paint the box a base color using acrylic paint, allow to dry and then, using a sea sponge, lightly touch the surface with a contrasting shade. Ivory or rose sponged with gold or powder blue with silver are especially nice. It's important to use a sea sponge because the holes in it make interesting patterns. In a pinch, you can use crumpled plastic wrap to dab the surface of your box with a contrasting color.

After applying a base coat of acrylic paint to a box you may stencil it with stars, hearts, leaves, or flowers. Or you can use Plaid's Decorator Color Blocks to decorate the surface.

I've been using Decorator Color Blocks for several years and find them easier to use than stencils. The blocks work on the same principle as a rubber stamp. They are shapes punched out of foam sheets to which you apply paint to be stamped on various surfaces such as paper, wood, or fabric. Unlike a stencil, you can create many different patterns and designs with ease because the foam shapes will bend to fit any contour. The paints which come with the blocks are non-toxic and clean up is simply a matter of soap and water. Check the source guide on page 153 for help finding these wonderful decorating tools.

DECORATING BOTTLES

Bottles offer lots of decorating possibilities. A pearl or antique button can be glued to the top of the cork or used to embellish the bottle itself. When you glue to glass, be sure to use an adhesive that is made to work with glass. Everyday white glue won't work.

Canning jars, which come in a variety of styles and sizes, are wonderful for packaging your bath salts and potpourri. To decorate a canning jar lid, take pinking shears and cut out a circle of fabric that is an inch larger in diameter than the lid. Apply white glue to the outer edge of the jar lid and place the fabric on top, smoothing it over the edges. When the glue dries, add a jute tie, a ribbon bow or some braid around the edge of the lid.

You can decorate the outside of a bottle with tulle, lace, silk, or a vintage handkerchief by folding it around a bottle and tying it with a cord and tassel. This fabric wrap can also be used to enclose a plastic bag of bath salts or potpourri.

Pretty ribbons and trims could also be used to add interest to a package. Tie them around the neck of your perfume bottle or add a bow to the top of a dusting powder container with hot glue or tacky glue. I also like to decorate with wired flowers and leaves. Start by trimming the bottle's neck with lace or ribbon. Then, using hot glue or thick, tacky glue, apply the flowers and leaves to the trim.

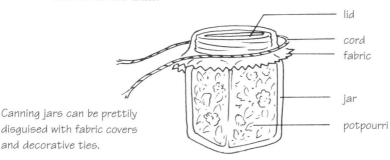

Canning jars can be prettily disguised with fabric covers and decorative ties.

lid

cord
fabric

jar

potpourri

Other Containers

Flowerpots can double as baskets for holding your gifts. Paint your flowerpot a soft aqua, then gild the edges of its rim with Rub 'n Buff, a metallic decorating finish. The pot can also be découpaged with paper or fabric cut-outs of flowers or perfume bottles and sealed with a clear acrylic spray.

You can use a decorative paper dinner napkin to cover your pot. Most of these napkins have two layers, a decorative layer backed by a white layer. Separate the two layers, discard the white backing then center the pot on the decorative portion of the napkin. Paint the pot with white craft glue and press the napkin up and over the lip of the pot. Allow to dry, then apply another thin coat of glue evenly over the outside of the pot. Fill the pot with colored tissue or excelsior and your scented gifts. If you use a decorated terra cotta pot for planting, insert a plastic liner before adding soil.

Cover an ordinary flowerpot with decorative paper or fabric.

DÉCOUPAGE, A FAVORITE PASTIME OF THE VICTORIANS

Apply a base coat of acrylic paint to the box or flower pot you wish to decorate. Cut out the design you would like to apply to the surface with small cuticle or embroidery scissors. Designs can be found in wrapping paper, seed and flower catalogs, dried flowers (as long as they are flat), calendars, fabric, postcards, or greeting cards. If you decide to use a postcard or greeting card, soak the backside of the card with water for a minute so that some of the paper can be peeled away. Otherwise, the card may be too thick. Make sure the card is dry before you continue.

Use a sponge or a sponge brush to apply a découpage coating to the back of the paper or fabric. I use Royal Coat or Mod Podge, available in craft stores, for my découpaging. Apply your design to the box or pot and use your fingers to smooth out any air bubbles.

Allow to dry for 30 minutes. Then apply two coats of découpage finish, allowing twenty minutes of drying time between coats.

If you want your finished piece to have an antiqued look, apply an antiquing stain (available at hardware and craft stores) after the first finish coat of découpage. Wipe it off with cheesecloth until your desired finish is achieved. Allow to dry for twenty minutes then apply your second finish coat of découpage medium.

FLOWER DECORATIONS

My favorite decorations are silk wired-ribbon flowers. They make any gift extra special. There are many beautiful colors and combinations of silk wired-ribbon. In addition to solid colored ribbons, ombré or shaded ones are available to make the blooms look even more realistic. Wired ribbon also comes in sheer organdy and moiré. Wired ribbon comes in widths such as #3 (⅝ inch), #5 (⅞ inch), #9 (1½ inch), and #40 (2¾ inch). See the source guide on page 153 for help finding wired ribbon.

Roses

1. Cut a 22-inch length of wired ribbon. A #9 (1½ inch) is the size I prefer to use.
2. Tie a knot in one end of the ribbon.
3. Pull the copper wire from one edge of the end opposite the knot, loosely gathering the ribbon along the wire until you reach the knot. Do not pull too hard as the wire is fragile and can break.

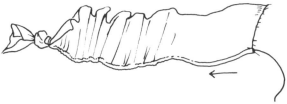

4. Continue gathering until the entire edge is ruffled and curling naturally. Leave the wire end free and DO NOT CUT OFF.
5. Holding the knot in one hand, begin to shape the rose by wrapping the ribbon around the knot. Wrap tightly at first to form a bud, then continue wrapping loosely so that the rose flares out into an open flower shape.

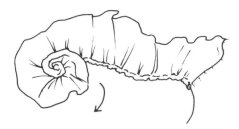

6. Fold the raw end down to meet the gathered edge, as shown by dotted line in the illustration below.

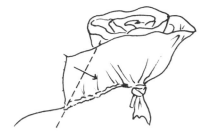

7. Secure rose by catching the free end with the wire and wrapping it tightly around the knot. Cut off any remaining wire.

8. Adjust rose petals as needed by ruffling or crinkling them.

Geraniums

Geraniums can be fashioned from wired or non-wired ribbon. If you use non-wired ribbon, you'll get your best results from two-sided satin or silk ribbon. Tricolored striped ribbon, such as peach, watermelon, and green make especially nice flowers of this type. Striped ribbon, pink and white for instance, will make these flowers look like petunias.

These directions are for non-wired ribbon. For wired ribbon instructions, please see above.

1. Cut a 12-inch length of #9 ribbon.

2. Knot the end of a 12-inch piece of matching thread and baste down the center of the ribbon from one end to the other.

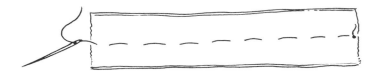

3. Pull on the loose end of the thread until the ribbon pleats itself into a ruffled bloom.

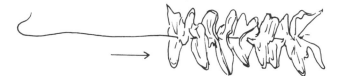

4. Knot off the thread and secure with a few stitches. Use these flowers singly with two leaves to create a petunia or sew several together for the look of a geranium in full bloom.

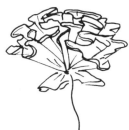

Leaves

Once you have fashioned a flower, make some leaves to go with it.

1. Cut a 5-inch piece of #5 (⅞ inch) wired ribbon. For a larger leaf, use #9 (½ inch) ribbon. Fold as shown below.
2. Fold again to form a point at the top.
3. Gather across the raw edges with wire or needle and thread to form a leaf.

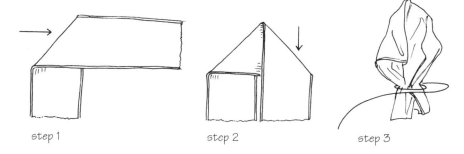

step 1   step 2   step 3

Kimono Leaves

The kimono-style leaf can be made with wired or unwired ribbon.

1. Cut a 2½- to 3-inch length of #9 (1½ inch) ribbon.
2. Find the midpoint and fold first the left then the right side down, forming a point.
3. Baste across the bottom, pull tight, and then knot off.

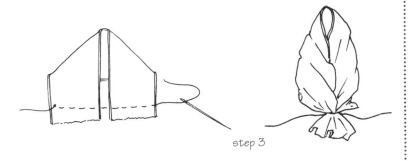

step 3

SCENTED GIFTS WITH A THEME

I love to take a pretty container and fill it with scented treasures. You can use a color theme for your gift based on the time of year or the recipient's favorite colors. In addition to your fragrances, roll up a washcloth or hand towel and tie it with a pretty ribbon; add a scented candle, or some wonderful soap.

And remember to always keep your eyes open for flea market finds such as teapots, sugar bowls, Depression glass, and glass salt or spice shakers. These make wonderful containers for dusting powder, potpourri, and bath salts.

PLEASE REMEMBER . . .

The joy of fragrance includes its ability to bring happy memories to mind and heart. So . . . "don't forget to smell the roses" and all the other wonderful fragrances in our beautiful world. Build yourself a garden of memories, never to be forgotten and always present to warm your heart.

Scentsationally yours,
Nancy M. Booth

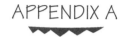
Perfumes Listed by Fragrance Family

WOMEN'S FRAGRANCES

SINGLE FLORAL

Carnation
Bellodgia

Gardenia
Gardenia Passion
Jungle Gardenia

Lily of the Valley
Diorissimo
Muguet des Bois

Narcissus
Narcisse Noir

Stephanotis
Nocturnes

Rose
Evelyn
Le Rose Jacqueminot
One Perfect Rose
Paris
Rose Absolue
Tea Rose

Tuberose
Blonde
Chloé
Fracas
Jontue
Phantom of the Opera
Tuberose

FLORAL BLENDS
Alfred Sung Forever
Amarige
Anne Klein
Antonia's Flowers East Hampton
Après L'Ondée
AV
Beautiful
Bill Blass
Blue Grass
Bulgari Eau Parfumée
Calla
Carolina Herrera
Catalyst
Champs Elysée
Chanel No. 22
Courrèges in Blue
Delicious
Destiny
Diamonds and Emeralds
Dilys
DNA
Donna Karan New York
Dream
Eau de Ciel
Elixir of Love No. 1
Ellen Tracy
Escada
Estée
Eternity
Fidji
Fleurs de Rocaille
Fleur d'Interdit
Flore

WOMEN'S FRAGRANCES (CONT'D.)

Floret
Fred Hayman's Touch
Gianfranco Ferre
Giorgio Beverly Hills
Golconda
Grand Amour
Habanita
Icewater
Jardins de Bagatelle
Je Reviens
Joy
K de Krizia
Kenzo
L'Aimant
L'Air du Temps
Laguna
Laura Biagiotti
Lalique
L'Heure Bleu
L'Interdit
Longing
Lumière
Mad Moments
Mariella Burani
Natori
Nicole Miller
Nine
Nocturnes
Norell (green)
No Regrets
Norma Kamali
Ombre Rose
1000 de Jean Patou
Oscar de la Renta
Passion
Passion Flower
Pavlova
Poême
Quadrille

Quelques Fleures L'Original (first
   true multi-floral)
Red Door
Red Jeans
Romeo Gigli
Scaasi
Society
So Pretty de Cartier
Sublime
Tatiana
Tendre Poison
360°
Tiffany
tommy girl
True Love
24 Faubourg
"273" for Women
Vanilla Fields
Vicky Tiel
Vivid
White Diamonds
White Rose
White Shoulders
Zinnia

FRUITY FLORALS
Amazone
Byblos
Champagne
Dalissimée
Design
Diamonds and
   Sapphires
Dolce Vita
Eau de Charlotte
Elysium
Escape
Ferre by Ferre
Gucci Accenti

WOMEN'S FRAGRANCES (CONT'D.)

Head Over Heels
Il Bacio
Issey Miyake
Jaipur de Boucheron
Jess
Joop! Pour Femme
Kashaya
Laura Ashley No. 1
Lauren
Listen
Liz Claiborne
Molinard de Molinard
Must de Cartier II
Nino Cerruti — 1881
Perry Ellis America for
   Women
Romeo Gigli
Senso
Smalto Donna
Sweet Courrèges
Trueste

**FLORAL ORIENTAL
(FLORIENTAL)**
Allure
Amber Antique
Asja
Bijan Perfume for
   Women
Bridges
Boucheron
Byzance
Chamade
Charles of the Ritz
Chloé Narcisse
Diamonds and Rubies
Di Borghese
Dolce & Gabanna
Escada
Fifth Avenue

First
Galanos
Galore
Hugo Boss Woman
Hanae Mori
Incognito
Jean Paul Gaultier
Jill Sanders No. 4
Joop! Pour Femme
Mackie
Marina De Bourbon
Navy
O de Lancôme
Panthère
Rapture
Realities
St. John
Samsara
Sirène Vicky Tiel
Spellbound
Sun, Moon, Stars
Trésor
Tuscany Per Donna
Van Cleef & Arpels
Vanderbilt
Venezia
Wings
. . . With Love

ORIENTAL
Bal à Versailles
Bijan
Black Pearls
Casmir
Chantilly
Chaos
Dioressence
Emeraude
Fath de Fath
Habanita

Insensé
L'Origan
Magie Noire
Must de Cartier
Nuit de Noël
Obsession
Opium
Parfum d'Hermès
Raffinée
Realm
Roma
Royal Secret
Shalimar
Shocking
Ugo Vanelli (fruity)
Vol de Nuit

CHYPRE
Animale
Aromatics Elixir
Azurée
Bandit
Cabochard
Calèche
Cassini
Chant d'Arômes
Coriandre
Crêpe de Chine
Cristalle
Cuir de Russie (leather
   notes)
Deci-Delà
Demi-Jour
Diva
Earth
Eau de Rochas
Féminité Du Bois
Femme
Fendi
Gem

WOMEN'S FRAGRANCES (CONT'D.)

Gianni Versace
Givenchy III
Gucci No. 3
Halston
Knowing
Ma Griffe
Miss Dior
Mitsouko (fruity)
Moments
Montana
Mystère de Rochas
Niki de St. Phalle
Paloma Picasso
Private Collection
V'E Versace
Wrappings
Ysatis

GREEN
Aliage
Amphibia
Cabotine
Calandre
Calyx
Chanel No. 19
Charlie
Eau de Camille
Eau de Givenchy
Envy
Giò
Grass
Jessica McClintock
Jicky (fougère)
K de Krizia
Parfum d'Eté (fougère)
Private Number
Safari
Sung
Vent Vert

CITRUS
Alfred Sung Spa
Amazone Eau de
  Fraicheur
Caron Eau de Cologne
Cristalie Eau de
  Parfum
Day
Eau de cologne
Eau de Guerlain
Eau d'Hadrien
Eau d'Hermès
Eau de Rochas
Eau Sauvage
Gieffeffe
Impériale
Jean Naté
Pitsenbon
Spring Fever
Verbena

OCEANIC
Acqua di Giò
Curve
Dune
Escada Acte 2
Escada Sport Scents
Fleur d'Eau
Gieffeffe
Giorgio Aire
Heaven (Gap)
L'Eau by Laura Ashley
  (tea notes)
L'Eau d'Issey
L'Eau De Monteil
New West Skinscent
  for Her
Ocean Dreams
Pleasures

Polo Sport for Women
Sunflowers
Tiffany Spa
tommy girl
Un Air de Samsara
White Linen Breeze
XS Pour Elle

SPICY
Angel
Ceylon
Cinnabar
Coco
KL
Ma Liberté
Organza
Parfum Sacré
Poison

MODERN ALDEHYDE
BLENDS
Antilope
Arpège
Calandre
Calèche
Chanel No. 5
Gucci No. 1
Infini
Le Dix
Liu
Lutèce
Madame Rochas
My Sin
Nahema
Red
Rive Gauche
Salvador Dali
White Linen

MEN'S FRAGRANCES

SPICY
Baryshnikov Pour Homme
Bijan for Men
Derby
DK Men Unleaded (herbaceous)
Eau de Lanvin
Egoïste (woody)
Francesco Smalto
Givenchy Gentlemen
Grès Monsieur
Herrera for Men
Homme Joop!
Ice Blue Aqua Velva
Jaguar
Montana Pour Homme
Newport
Old Spice
Royall Bay Rhum
Royall Spyce
Rugger
Sables
Salvador
Santes de Cartier

CITRUS
America for Men
Armani pour Homme
Blue Jeans
Boucheron
Catalyst
Dolce & Gabanna for Men (citrus-woody)
Drakkar
Dunhill for Men (floral)
Eau de Rochas (green)
Eau de Givenchy
Eau Sauvage

Eau Sauvage Extrême
Escape for Men (woodsy-fougère)
Fendi Uomo
Green Water
Gucci Nobile
Habit Rouge
Heaven (amber)
Héritage
Insatiable
Jill Sanders Feeling Man
KL Homme (amber)
L'eau d'Issey for Men
M for Men
Mackie for Men
Metropolis
Nautica (oceanic)
Santos Eau de Sport
Tiffany (woody-citrus)
tommy

LAVENDER
Aqua Lavanda
Lavande
Le Male
Old English Lavender
Old Spice Fresh Scent
Pino Silvestre (conifer)
Pour un Homme
Ungara Pour Homme I

WOODY
Acqua di Giò for Men
Aramis
Bill Blass
Boss Elements
Cerruli Pour Homme
Cool Water (fruity)

Eternity (fruity)
Fahrenheit
Gianfranco Ferre for Men
Giorgio Beverly Hills for Men
Halston 101
HUGO
Kenzo pour Homme (green)
Lauder for Men
Minotaure
Night Flight (fruity)
Patou pour Homme
Photo (fruity)
Red for Men
Safari for Men
Sybaris
Tricorn
Tuscany Forte
Versace L'Homme
Vetiver
Xeryus
Xeryus Rouge pour Homme (green)

FOUGÈRE
Arden for Men
Azzaro Pour Homme
Basala
Boss
Brut for Men
Calvin
Canoe
Chaps
Devin
Drakkar Noir
Egoïste Platinum
Havana

MEN'S FRAGRANCES (CONT'D.)

Lacoste
L'Homme
Paco Rabanne
Patou pour Homme
   Privé (amber-floral)
Scott McClintock
Smalto
Ungaro III
Wings for Men
YSL

ORIENTAL
Bulgari Pour Homme
Escada Pour Homme
Opium for Men
Obsession for Men
Realm for Men

LEATHER
Antaeus
Bel Ami
DK Men
English Leather
Knize Ten
Lanvin for Men
Pour Lui
Quorum
Royal Copenhagen

CHYPRE
Animale for Men
Cassini
Chanel Pour Monsieur
Chevignon (green)
Dali pour Homme

Davidoff
Elements
Escada for Men
Grés Pour Homme
Grey Flannel (green)
Halston Limited
JHL
Kouros
New West for Him
Oscar Pour Lui
Polo (green)
Polo Crest
Quorum
Ungaro Pour Homme

UNISEX FRAGRANCES

Bel Amis
Bulgari Eau Parfumée
   (green tea)

cK one (floral)
cK be (musk)
Eau d'Hadrian

Eau Sauvage
Paco (citrus)

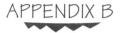
Perfumers and Their Perfumes

With so many perfumers and scents, it is impossible to include all of them in this book. I've chosen some of the more important noses (and their fragrances), however, so you will have more information about perfume. I've also included the top, middle, and base notes of each fragrance in its description so that if you enjoy the scent of Anaïs Anaïs or Red Door, you can try your hand at creating a fragrance at home that will resemble your favorite perfume.

Arden — Elizabeth Arden's sweet floral Blue Grass (1935), the favorite perfume of Queen Elizabeth II, was named for the view from the windows of Arden's Virginia home. Her Red Door is a saucy floral composed of red roses, jasmine, lily of the valley, and rare winter-blooming oriental orchids mingled with freesias, wild violets, and a finishing touch of vetiver and a hint of honey.

Armani — Fashion designer Giorgio Armani's Giò (pronounced "Joe") arrived in 1993. It is composed of green, fruit-floral top notes, and a true hyacinth fragrance, a hint of peach, and heart notes of jasmine, gardenia, tuberose, and orange blossom warmly based in vanilla, amber, and woody notes. Acqua di Giò (1995), one of my favorite anytime fragrances, is a transparent scent based on marine notes, fresh florals, and sweet peas on a musky wood base.

Ashley — Laura Ashley's beautiful glass flacons are etched with flowers in several hues and contain Laura Ashley No. 1 (1989), a soft, fruity, floral with top notes of peach, gardenia, hyacinth, and bergamot, heart notes of narcissus, rose, jasmine, orchid, clove, and carnation with undertones of musk, vanilla, cyclamen, and sandalwood. It is a truly romantic scent not unlike her wonderful fabrics and fashions.

Bellanca — Antonia Bellanca of East Hampton, New York, is the creator of Antonia's Flowers (1984), inspired by memories of her grandmother's garden. Antonia combined freesias and jasmine with the delicious aromas of magnolias, lilies, and fruity notes encircling floral accords. This fragrance has a loyal following and is quite delightful.

Boucheron — Parfums Boucheron's Boucheron Classic (1988) is a warm and sensuous bouquet of semi-oriental floral notes. It is packaged in an exquisite bottle, designed by the jeweler of the same name, resembling a cabochon sapphire set in a ring of gold.

Bulgari — Bulgari, a world-renowned jeweler whose flagship store is in Rome, composed Bulgari Eau Parfumée (1993) with top notes of bergamot, orange blossom, cardamom, pepper, and coriander centered around Bulgarian rose and Egyptian jasmine and unusual base notes of woods and essence of green tea. Tea inspired Bulgari to create this perfume because this popular beverage symbolizes "time for a break, relaxation, and meditation."

Cacherel — French couturier Jean Bousquet, founder of Cacherel, describes his fragrance in these words: "Anaïs Anaïs (Persian goddess of love) is a perfume whose essence is romanticism with the scent of lilies." A feminine, youthful, and delicate fragrance, Anaïs Anaïs is packaged in a snow white opaline glass bottle bearing a peachy pink and celadon green label in a floral print from the textile designer Liberty of London. Madonna lilies, a symbol of purity to the Greeks and Romans, are the heart of this perfume. It takes one ton of petals to produce a pound of lily oil. Anaïs Anaïs has been a best-selling fragrance since its 1978 introduction.

Caron — The renowned perfumes of Caron began in 1903 when Ernest Daltroff opened this perfume house. Narcisse Noir (1911) established the brilliance of Caron with its notes of rose, jasmine, and orange blossom.

Cartier — A famous jeweler, Jacques Cartier expanded his horizons to perfume when he successfully introduced So Pretty de Cartier. There are three noteworthy elements in this special fragrance — centifolia rose, Florentine iris, and the Diamond orchid from Brazil. The rose blooms only in May and a single bottle of this perfume contains the essence of twelve thousand petals. The iris is the most expensive ingredient in perfumery today and the rare orchid's fragrance is released into the air only fifty minutes before twilight, making its extraction a delicate process.

Carven — Mme. Carven, a French couturier, is famous for Ma Griffe (1946), a romantic floral chypre, as well as her own personal fragrance. A favorite of Barbara Walters, this classic scent is an earthy blend of green notes, mosses, flowers, woods, and musk.

Chopard — Popular in Europe, Casmir (1991) was brought to the American market by the Lancaster Group in 1994. Chopard is also a jeweler of distinction and his fragrance is a fruity oriental with the exotic richness of vanilla, sandalwood, and patchouli coupled with lively mango, peach, and coconut. Chopard's Heaven (1995) is a bright citrus-amber.

Claiborne — After ten years as an American fashion designer, Liz Claiborne introduced her namesake perfume in 1986. A crisp and sporty blend, this fruity floral springs to life with a light floral accord and warm woody base notes that include green notes, white lily, mandarin, peach, and tagetes (marigold).

Crabtree & Evelyn — Evelyn (1993) is this firm's first eau de parfum. Although the singular impression is one of roses, eighty-five ingredients make up this fragrance. English rose grower David Austin developed this scent over an eight year period working with master perfumer V. Mane of Grasse, France. Living flower technology was employed to create an exact rendition of the Evelyn rose for this perfume.

De La Renta — Oscar de la Renta's Oscar (1978) is a floral-amber perfume inspired by his mother's gardens of fragrant white blossoms native to his Dominican Republic. Fruit and spice top notes with a heady blend of tuberose, rose de mai, jasmine, and ylang-ylang are warmed with a woody accord of myrrh, opopanax, cloves, patchouli, lavender, and sandalwood.

Dior — Christian Dior founded the House of Dior in 1947 and came out with Miss Dior the same year. This perfume is a green floral with chypre, sage, gardenia, galbanum, rose, jasmine, neroli, patchouli, and labdanum. In 1956, perfumer Edmond Roudnitska called Dior's Diorissimo "a pure lily of the valley scent that also has the odor of the woods in which it is found and the indefinable atmosphere of springtime."

Ellis — Perry Ellis's 360° (1993) is a clear, bright combination of Amazon lily, osmanthus, living melon, tangerine, and blue rose. Its heart is a rich, white, floral bouquet of muguet, water lily, and lavender with a touch of sage. Amber, sandalwood, vetiver, vanilla, and musk form the base notes.

Erox Corporation — Realm for Women (1993) is an oriental scent and the first to contain synthesized human pheromones. Pheromones are organic scent signals used to communicate. The word pheromone comes from the Greek words pherein (to carry) and hormon (to excite). Top notes begin with Sicilian mandarin, Italian cassia, and Egyptian tagetes that continue with fresh living peony and water lilies. Its warm, sensual drydown includes sandalwoods warmed by honey and vanilla.

Givenchy — Hubert de Givenchy, a French couturier, made a perfume especially for Audrey Hepburn called L'Interdit (the forbidden one) and used her lovely visage to launch it to the public in 1957. Ysatis, a chypre floral and complex best-selling fragrance, arrived in 1985. Its top notes of mandarin, coconut, bergamot, ylang ylang, greens, and rosewood have a central theme of rose, iris, tuberose, jasmine, narcissus, and carnation. Warm base notes include oakmoss, vetiver, patchouli, bay rum, vanilla, clove, honey, and civet.

Goutal — Annick Goutal is a well-regarded French perfumer whose fragrances are meant to be mixed and layered. Passion (1986) is a sensual, heady blend of tuberose, jasmine, and vanilla. It is long-lasting floral scent, totally feminine and luxurious. Rose Absolue is a mélange of six varieties of roses: Bulgarian, May, Turkish, Damask, Egyptian, and Moroccan. Eau d' Hadrien is a refreshingly tart, citrusy blend of Sicilian lemon, grapefruit, citron, and cypress and can be worn by both men and women seeking a sporty, active scent equally at home on the tennis court or going out to brunch. Gardenia Passion embodies the memorable scent of these creamy blooms.

Halston — The signature fragrance, Halston, is a chypre-floral blend of green notes followed by fruity essences and a floral bouquet supported by an amber base.

Haymen — Gale and Fred Haymen's Giorgio (1982) was named after their Rodeo Drive boutique in Beverly Hills. An impressive fragrance and one of the best sellers ever known, it is a heady floral centered around jasmine, rose, carnation, gardenia, orangeflower, chamomile, sandalwood, and patchouli.

Kenzo — Kenzo, a Japanese designer, came out with Parfum d'Été, a vibrant and warm scent like a beautiful summer day. Fragrant accords of green leaves, sap, rose, peony, jasmine, and a rare tropical flower rise and blossom in the sun. Kashaya arrived in 1996 with top notes of apricot, hyacinth, rose, and "living" elementine developed with headspace technology designed to accurately replicate the scent of living plants.

Lagerfeld — Karl Lagerfeld, a haute couture designer, produces Chloe, which originally appeared in 1975. The main body of this scent is a heady tuberose, an aroma that is unforgettable. There are also notes of jasmine, orangeflower, and honeysuckle. Sun, Moon, Stars, another Lagerfeld fragrance, is a modern floral with oriental overtones. Sun-loving heliotrope is at the heart of the composition along with night-blooming jasmine, orange blossom, and narcissus. The vibrant base notes include sandalwood, amber, and musk.

Lancôme — Lancôme was founded by Armand Petitjean in 1935. Trésor, one of the top ten best-selling perfumes in the world since its introduction in 1991, blends rose, muguet, lilac, and apricot blossoms with middle notes of heliotrope and iris and base notes of sandalwood, amber, and musk.

Lauren — American designer Ralph Lauren's fresh, feminine Lauren was launched in 1978. It is a fruity floral, a timeless classic of green notes and wild marigolds, with a heart of jonquil, violet, muguet, Bulgarian rose, and jasmine floating on a base of carnation and vetiver, delicately balanced with warm woods and exotic spices.

Ley — Magaretha Ley, a Swedish designer, brought out Escada in 1990. This floriental scent has top notes of bergamot, hyacinth from the south of France, and a bouquet of peach and coconut. The heart notes are jasmine, ylang-ylang, orangeflower, and orris, resting on a base of Madagascar vanilla and Indian sandalwood against a background of powdery musk.

Miglin — Marilyn Miglin's Pheromone (1980) has a very interesting story attached to it which she was kind enough to share. After researching the history of perfume, Marilyn learned that in the early Egyptian civilization certain scents were considered more precious than gold. In Egypt, she discovered perfume recipes etched in hieroglyphics on stone walls. An Egyptologist deciphered the writings containing the secrets of the ancient perfumes. The perfumer Ms. Miglin contacted on her return to New York was amazed at the sophistication of methods employed over five thousand years ago. Pheromone is a balanced blend of 179 rare and costly essences, combining full-bodied florals, exotic green notes, spices, and woody notes. Her fragrance Magic has a "mysterious quality of enchantment" with top notes of Belgian cassis, jasmine, Moroccan sweet almond oil, and bergamot from Calabria. The heart notes are heliotrope and tuberose. Vanilla, geranium, and plum make up the base notes.

Miller — Nicole Miller's signature scent of the same name is called an aura-floral, a new concept in perfumery, designed to drape a fragrant silhouette over the entire body. Mandarin and peach top notes wrap around a floral core softened with woody accords.

Millot — Millot was established in the nineteenth century and was most famous for the creation of Crêpe de Chine (1925), a floral chypre with a powdery veil of fragrance. Jean Desprez, its creator, went on to fashion Bal à Versailles in 1962. Its composition of jasmine and rose and orange blossom create the initial impression; at the heart are spicy accords of sandalwood, patchouli, and vetiver, with the lasting qualities of musk, civet, and ambergris.

Miyake — In 1992, Issey Miyake introduced L'Eau d'Issey, a dewy, aquatic scent, punctuated with verdant green notes, a flowery heart of peony, white lilies, and a touch of spicy carnation. This fruity floral is fresh, crisp and a wonderful scent for casual, sporty, daytime wear.

Mugler — Thierry Mugler's Angel (1992) is a wonderful example of a spicy oriental scent with top notes of dewberry, green and fruity notes, and honey with a delectable heart of chocolate and caramel finished with vanilla and patchouli. Mugler says that the scent is meant to "stir child-hood memories." His personal symbol is the star, and Angel's flacon is of crystal blue in the shape of a five pointed star.

Penhaligon — In 1870, William Henry Penhaligon opened a barber shop in London and soon produced a jasmine and sandalwood scent called Hammam Bouquet. Its popularity helped him to become the toast of London society. To honor Sir Winston Churchill, who was born at Blenheim Palace in Oxfordshire, Penhaligon created Blenheim Bouquet, a blend of lime and pine which remains their best seller today.

St. Laurent — Opium by Yves St. Laurent zoomed into the marketplace in 1977 and was an instant success. Opium is a warm oriental fragrance of myrrh, benzoin, and sandalwood, with floral notes of carnation, rose, lily of the valley, and jasmine. The fruity top notes of plum are spiced with pepper, clove, and coriander. Opium for Men arrived in 1996, a fresh oriental whose predominent note is vanilla. It has top notes of black currant and star anise. The spicy heart combines the gingery scent of Chinese galganga and szechuan pepper. The warm and woody base notes of atlas cedar and tolu balsam give the fragrance a unique signature. Those who love roses should definitely try Yves St. Laurent's Paris.

Schiaparelli — Elsa Schiaparelli, a surrealist fashion designer of the 1930s, collaborated with Salvador Dali when she brought out her sweet, oriental perfume, Shocking. She had chosen a bright, hot pink for the packaging and it occurred to her while searching for a name how outrageous the color she had chosen was; hence the name Shocking. Her shade of pink would also become known by this name. During the fashion season of 1937, it was a very popular hue indeed.

Sung — Alfred Sung, an international designer, has a lovely white, floral fragrance called Sung (1986). The scent is fresh and light, alive with green citrus notes against a background of woods and spices. The top notes are mandarin, ylang-ylang, galbanum, lemon, hyacinth, followed by osmanthus, jasmine, iris, and lily of the valley, finished with vanilla, orange blossom, sandalwood, amber, and vetiver.

Tiffany — Tiffany perfume was created to honor the store's 150th anniversary in 1987. This sophisticated yet romantic fragrance is a floral-amber blend, with top notes of Indian jasmine, Damascene rose, ylang-ylang, mandarin, and orangeblossom. The central theme is iris, black currant buds, and violet leaves and the base notes are sandalwood, amber, vanilla, and vetiver.

Van Cleef & Arpels — Parisian jewelers Van Cleef & Arpels introduced First in 1976, a floral bouquet enhanced with sparkling, aldehydic notes and warmed with a sweet amber and wood base. Their scent Van Cleef & Arpels (1993) is available only in perfume and eau de parfum. It is a floriental with herbs, fruits and spices as top notes, a heart of rose, jasmine, jonquil, and mimosa absolute, rounded out with vanilla, musk, cedarwood, and tonka bean.

APPENDIX C

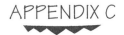

Fragrant Flowers and Their Scents

Many people complain that flowers "just don't smell the way they used to." The flowers listed below are among the many antique — and fragrant — blooms being preserved by nurseries all over the country. And the sources for these heavenly flowers are listed at the end of this appendix. If you're going to grow flowers, grow the kind that fill the air with fragrance.

Drying Flowers

There are several ways to dry flowers. You can put them in the microwave for one to four minutes, depending on their density. I prefer to dry them naturally, however, in order to preserve their color better. Dry rose heads and petals on paper towels in a warm, dry place such as the kitchen, attic, or garage. They must be dried in a single layer so they will not mildew.

Flowers can also be dried by hanging them upside down, also in a warm, dry place. Secure the stems with a tight rubber band which will shrink as the flowers dry. You can hang them from a length of heavy string or clothesline by hooking a paper clip through the rubber band and then onto the line.

Flowers may also be dried and pressed flat between pieces of blotter paper weighted down by heavy books or another appropriate weight. When selecting flowers for drying, take the following into consideration: white flowers tend to turn brown when drying and dark red flowers turn black while drying.

ROSES

Variety	Scent	Color
Hybrid Tea		
Color Magic	china tea	shades of pink
Fragrant Cloud	tangerine-orange	red-orange
French Perfume	apples and berries	pink
Fortune Teller	lemon-honey	deep pink
Heirloom	fruity	deep lilac
Just Joey	fruity rose	apricot

Variety	Scent	Color
Hybrid Tea (cont'd.)		
Legend	peach-pear	red
Perfume Delight	sweet rose	pink
Sutter's Gold	fruity	yellow
Tropicana	raspberry-lime	coral-orange
Grandiflora		
Arizona	strong tea rose	copper gold
Sonia	spicy	peach
Floribunda		
Angel Face	old-fashioned rose	lavender
Apricot Nectar	fruity	apricot
Intrigue	lemony	red-purple
Love Potion	raspberry	lavender
Bourbon		
Honorine de le Brabant	raspberry	pale pink splashed with purple and crimson
La Reine Victoria	heady rose	violet
Mme. Ernst Calvet	old-fashioned rose	clear pink
Mme. Isaac Pereire	raspberry	crimson pink
Souvenir de Malmaison	spicy	soft pink
Moss		
Salet	musk	powder pink
Centifolia		
Fantin Latour	soft rose	pink
Alba		
Maiden's Blush	delicate rose	pale pink
Portland		
Jacques Cartier	old-fashioned rose	dark pink

ENGLISH ROSES BY DAVID AUSTIN

*Evelyn	old rose	delicious rose pink
Gertrude Jekyll	heavy rose	deep pink
Golden Celebration	honey	sunshine yellow
Graham Thomas	lime, cinnamon, clove	golden yellow

*Evelyn was developed by David Austin for Crabtree and Evelyn's rose fragrance of the same name.

LILACS

Variety	Color
Ami Schott	lavender
Katherine Havemeyer	mauve pink
Ludwig Spaeth	reddish purple
Victor Le Moine	rosy pink

SWEET VIOLETS

Coeur d'Alsace	rose pink
Princess of Wales	violet blue
Royal Robe	deep purple

LAVENDER

L. angustifolia	lavender blue
L. spica	soft lavender

GARDENIA (do not dry well; only for use in fragrance crafting)

August Beauty	ivory
Mystery	ivory

SWEET PEAS

America	striped red
Crimson Excelsior	crimson
Cupani	deep maroon, purple (named for the Italian monk who discovered sweet peas)
Cuthbertson's Mix	multicolored mix
Elizabeth Taylor	lavender
Geranium Pink	deep pink
Leamington	lilac to lavender
Noel Sutton	rich mid-blue
Old Spice	cream pink, rose lavender, rich purple
Picadilly	salmon to rose red
Painted Lady	delicate pink

PANSIES*

Variety	Color
Imperial ntique	peach, gold, and rose
Love Duet	rose and cream
Maxim Marina	blue, lavender, and white
Watercolor Mix	range of soft pastels

Not for fragrance, but easy to press between the pages of a book (I use my phone book) for color and to decorate your final creations.

Sources for Fragrant Plants and Flowers

Note: Be sure to check and see which varieties will perform best in your zone and climate.

Antique Rose Emporium
800-441-0002
www.antiqueroseemporium.com

Jackson & Perkins
800-872-7673
www.jacksonandperkins.com

Renee's Garden Seeds
888-880-7228
www.reneesgarden.com

Sandy Mush Herb Nursery
828-683-2014
www.sandymushherbs.com
Wonderful selection of scented geraniums and herbs

Select Seeds - Antique Flowers
800-684-0395
www.selectseeds.com

Thompson & Morgan
800-274-7333
www.thompson-morgan.com
Many types of pansies and a wonderful selection of fragrant sweet peas

Wayside Gardens
800-213-0379
www.waysidegardens.com

White Flower Farm
800-503-9624
www.whiteflowerfarm.com

SOURCE GUIDE

Kits

To make it easier for you to start your fragrance crafting, you can use the following kits by Gingham 'n' Spice. Each kit includes:

4 ounces rosewater
4 ounces jojoba oil
4 ounces glycerin
2 droppers
2 ½-ounce glass bottles with glass rods attached to tops
6 ⅛-ounce vials of fragrance or essential oils (see below)

A) Floral Bouquet / Fruity Floral
pear • peach • cinnamon
rose • gardenia • vanilla

B) Oriental / Floriental
petitgrain • heliotrope • rose
stephanotis • honeysuckle • vanilla

C) Woodsy / Spicy
clovebud • allspice • bergamot
lavender • bay • cedarwood

D) Green / Chypre
nutmeg • lavender • violet
hyacinth • chypre • cedarwood

E) Citrus / Cologne / Floral
rose • sweet orange • lemon
verbena • lavender • bergamot
clovebud

Order at:

My Sweet Victoria
267-354-1362
www.fragrancesupplies.com

Other Supplies

Alban Muller International
305-994-7558
www.albanmuller.com
Herbal extracts, oils, and butters

Arista Industries, Inc.
800-255-6457
www.aristaindustries.com
Carrier oils (such as jojoba, almond, and apricot kernel)

Aura Cacia
800-437-3301
www.auracacia.com
Essential and fragrance oils

Aveda
866-823-1425
www.aveda.com
Essential and fragrance oils

C. M. Offray and Son
800-344-5533
www.offray.com
Wired ribbon

Camden-Grey Essential Oils
888-207-9724
www.camdengrey.com

Colorful Images
800-458-7999
www.colorfulimages.com
Small runs of labels which can
be ordered with your scented
creation's name or "handmade by"
and your name

Country Herbals by Andrea
570-996-0910
www.countryherbals.com
Handmade soaps

**E. D. Luce Prescription
Packaging**
562-802-0515
www.essentialsupplies.com
Wholesale bottles, vials, jars,
and apothecary supplies

Essence of Life
505-758-7941
www.sacredoilsofkrishna.com
Indian aromatics

The Essential Oil Company
800-729-5912
www.essentialoil.com
Essential and fragrance oils

From Nature With Love
800-520-2060
www.fromnaturewithlove.com
Essential oils, floral waters, alcohol-
free fragrance oils, and more

Frontier Co-Op Herbs
800-669-3275
www.frontiercoop.com
Carrier oils (jojoba, sweet almond,
and apricot kernel), vanilla beans

**International Flavors &
Fragrances**
212-765-5500
www.iff.com
Fragrance oils

Kiehl's Pharmacy
800-543-4572
www.kiehls.com
Perfumes, natural bath and
body products

Lebermuth Company
800-648-1123
www.lebermuth.com
Carrier oils, essential and
fragrance oils

Lipo Chemicals
973-345-8600
www.lipochemicals.com
Carrier oils, glycerin

Milky Way Molds
503-482-5056
www.milkywaymolds.com
Soap molds

O. Berk Co.
908-851-9500
www.oberk.com
Bottles

Pier 1 Imports
800-245-4595
www.pier1.com

Plaid Enterprises
800-842-4197
www.plaidonline.com
Decorator Blocks®

Purcell Natural Jojoba
800-676-1501
www.purcelljojoba.com
Jojoba oil

Quilter's Resource
800-676-6543
www.quiltersresource.com
Wired ribbon

Ruger Chemical Co.
800-274-7843
www.rugerchemical.com
Glycerin

Samara Bontane
800-782-4532
www.wingedseed.com
Essential oils and accessories

Sensory Essence
847-526-3645
www.organicbulgarianrose.com
Bulgarian aromatics

SKS Bottle & Packaging
518-880-6980
www.sks-bottle.com

Sunburst Bottle Company
916-929-4500
www.sunburstbottle.com
Bottles

Sun Feather Natural Soap
315-265-3648
www.sunfeather.com
Soap

Thornley Company
302-224-8300
www.thornleycompany.com
Carrier oils

Welch, Holme & Clark Co.
973-465-1200
www.welch-holme-clark.com
Carrier oils

Woodspirits Ltd.
937-663-4327
www.woodspirits.com
Handmade soap

RELATED READING MATERIAL

Cunningham, Scott. *The Complete Book of Incense, Oils and Brews.* St. Paul, MN: Llewellyn Publications, 1989.

Fettner, Ann Tucker. *Potpourri, Incense and Other Fragrant Concoctions.* New York: Workman Publishing Company, 1977.

Barille, Elisabeth and Catherine Laroze. *The Book of Perfume.* New York: Abbeville Press, 1995.

Riggs, Maribeth. *The Scented Woman.* New York: Penguin Books, 1992.

Irvine, Susan. *Perfume.* New York: Crescent Books, 1995.

The following books are a bit more difficult to find since some are out of print or specialized. If you're interested in researching more about the history and nature of perfume, these books are worth searching for in a library or from the publishers.

Groom, Nigel. *The Perfume Handbook.* New York: Chapman Hall, 1992.

Kennett, Frances. *History of Perfume.* London: Harrap, 1975.

Morris, Edwin T. *Fragrance, The Story of Perfume from Chanel to Cleopatra.* New York: Scribner, 1984.

Kauffman, William I. *Perfume.* New York: E.P. Dutton & Co., 1974.

The Fragrance and Olfactory Dictionary. New York: The Fragrance Foundation, 1994.

The Male Fragrance Adventure. New York: The Fragrance Foundation, 1995.

The History, the Mystery, the Enjoyment of Fragrance. New York: The Fragrance Foundation.

GLOSSARY

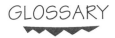

For fragrant ingredients, please see Chapter 2.

absolute — the most concentrated form of perfumery material usually obtained by alcohol extraction of concretes.

accord — a perfume composed of different scents which create a new fragrance composition when blended together.

aldehyde — ingredient in the manufacture of synthetic modern perfumes. The use of aldehydes in perfumes was a development of Ernest Beaux for Chanel No. 5, the first aldehydic fragrance. These fragrances have a rich and sparkling top note.

animalic — of animal origin, such as musk, civet, ambergris, and castoreum.

aroma chemicals — (1) nature-identical aroma chemicals; (2) chemicals isolated from natural origins; (3) synthetic aroma chemicals not found in nature but an important addition contributing unique odors.

aromacology — the study of the psychological effects of scents. Supported by the Olfactory Research Fund, uses psychology and fragrance technology and studies how odors transmit a variety of feelings to the right side of the brain or limbic system, the seat of emotions, memory, and creativity.

attar — also known as otto; essential oil obtained during distillation, in particular that of the Bulgarian Rose.

base notes — the underlying ingredients of fragrance, responsible for its lasting qualities. The ingredients used in base notes are often referred to as fixatives.

baudruchage — a method for sealing perfume flacons still employed by a few top perfume houses such as Patou (Joy). The neck of the perfume bottle is covered with a thin natural membrane (often pig's intestine), then tied with a cotton thread knotted four times to ensure an airtight seal.

beeswax — wax produced by honey bees, used in cosmetics and ointments.

blotter strip — a thin strip of absorbent filter paper used to evaluate a fragrance. Also called a mouillette.

bouquet — a well-rounded blend of two or more fragrance complexes. A dominant theme that expresses well-known flower types.

Carmelite water — a toilet water composed of orangeflower water, angelica root, lemon balm, and spices first prepared in 1379 by the nuns of the Carmelite abbey of St. Juste for Charles V of France.

cassolette — a box designed to hold a perfumed paste, having a perforated lid and usually made of ivory, gold, or silver.

chromatography — a method of scientific analysis used to determine the extent of an individual molecule's presence in a fragrance. Sometimes used to counterfeit well-known perfumes.

chypre — a perfume family originated in 1917 with François Coty's Chypre. Oakmoss, patchouli, labdanum, bergamot, calamus, clary sage, sandalwood, and vetiver are typical components in a chypre blend.

citrus notes — usually found in top notes and imparting a sharp, tangy scent. Citrus scents include lemon, lime, tangerine, mandarin, and bitter orange blossoms.

coconut oil — a white, semisolid fat that lathers well and is useful as a moisturizer or to blend with other oils. It melts when brought to room temperature.

concrete — a semisolid, waxy substance obtained by the extraction of essential oils by volatile solvents. Represents the closest odor duplication of the flower, bark, or leaves from which it has been extracted. Concretes can be further concentrated to produce absolutes.

Damask water — a perfume compound made from damask roses, popular in England during the sixteenth century.

diffusion — the ability of a fragrance to surround the wearer with an aura of scent.

distillation — a method of extracting essential oils using steam. Flowers and plants are submerged in boiling water and the resulting steam is then cooled. At this point the oil separates from the water and can be collected.

distilled water — water free of foreign substances; should be used in all fragrance recipes calling for water. Tap water contains additives and chemicals that can cause an adverse reaction in a blend.

dramming — a technique for transfering a fragrance from a larger to a smaller container.

dry perfume — a fragrance delivery system of essential fragrance oil micro-encapsulated in an alcohol-free pressed powder containing up to 25 percent oil. A portable, non-spill fragrance alternative.

drydown — the final phase of a fragrance as it develops on the skin. Perfumers evaluate the base notes and a fragrance's tenacity during this stage.

dry note — a woody and mossy note in a perfume blend.

earthy note — a note evoked by vetiver and patchouli.

eau de Cologne — a fragrance compound developed in Italy in the seventeenth century and commercially successful at the end of the eighteenth century in Cologne, Germany. A 2 percent to 5 percent ratio of perfume oils in a 70 percent alcohol/water mix.

eau de parfum — a fragrance compound containing an 8 to 15 percent concentration of oils diluted in 90-proof alcohol.

eau de toilette — a perfume oil concentration of 4 to 8 percent in an alcohol base.

eau fraîche — a toilet water made with a high grade of alcohol and a perfume oil concentration of 1 to 3 percent. The lightest form of fragrance.

enfleurage — a method, originating in ancient Eygpt, for extracting flower oil through the use of cold purified fats. The resulting pomade is put into an alcoholic solvent from which the fragrant oil is extracted. This method is very costly but produces the finest jasmine and tuberose oils. Rose, violet, jonquil, and mignonette oils are obtained through enfleurage as well.

essential oil — the essence of plants; the fragrant, volatile extracts obtained from flowers, grasses, seeds, leaves, roots, barks, fruits, mosses, and resins. Essential oils are the basic ingredients used by the perfumer.

expression — a method of obtaining essences used mainly to extract oils from citrus fruit rinds. The zest contains the scented oils, which are expressed using a hydraulic press.

extraction — the method most often used to obtain the oils of fragrant ingredients. Flower petals, leaves, etc. are added to volatile solvents at a low temperature. The solvents release the oils without the use of harmful heat. The solvent is then evaporated to obtain the concrete. A further process allows the alcohol to evaporate; the result is an absolute.

extrait — the most concentrated form of perfume. It is obtained through extraction using volatile solvents.

fixative — substances that modify the evaporation rate and prolong the continuity of the odor. Most often derived from mosses, resins, and aroma chemicals.

flacon — a small perfume bottle with an ornamental stopper designed to form an airtight seal.

floral note — present in all perfumes for men and women.

fougère — the French word for fern, describing notes of lavender, bergamot, oakmoss, and coumarin. Many popular men's fragrances fall into this category.

fragrance — an attractive scent, from the Latin *fragrare* (to smell).

fragrance oil — a combination of essential oils with added chemicals and fixed oils.

fragrance wardrobe concept — an idea conceived by The Fragrance Foundation in the early 1960s suggesting to the consumer that a wardrobe of a minimum of three to four fragrances allows one to express various moods, occasions, and fashions. The fragrance wardrobe might contain a floral bouquet, oriental, woodsy-mossy, and green type of scent.

fruity note — scents of ripe fruit and berries (excluding citrus) used in gourmand perfumes within their fragrance themes.

glycerin — from coconuts, seals in moisture and is beneficial for all skin types. An ingredient in lotions, creams, and soaps. Has the ability to make bubles and increase suds. Also used as a fixative in perfumes. Glycerin is known for its skin softening properties.

gourmand — having notes of ripe fruit, chocolate, honey, vanilla, caramel, and spice.

Grasse — a region in Provence in the south of France, the center of the French perfume industry since the sixteenth century. Famous too for the glorious flowers growing there.

green note — usually appearing as a top note, part of a family of scents with dewy, leafy aromas and the scents of newly mown grass.

hayfield notes — tones provided by coumarin and imbuing a perfume with the scent of new-mown hay.

headspace technology — the use of gas chromatography to map a fingerprint of odors in the air. Since flowers are still living and uncut during this process, the result is a perfect scent copy. Also called living flower technology.

herbaceous — having a fragrance note with a spicy, grassy green quality. Rosemary, lavender, and thyme are examples of herbaceous scents.

hesperides — a fragrance obtained from citrus fruits.

honey water — a toilet water popular in France and England since the eighteenth century.

incense — the original form in which fragrance was used. Combinations of resins, fragrant woods, and gums in solid or powdered forms which are burned to create an aromatic smoke. In ancient times, thought to be a pathway to heaven for prayers and therefore used extensively during religious ceremonies.

indole — a chemical occurring naturally in a number of essential oils such as jasmine, neroli, and orange blossom. Heavy florals are often referred to as indolic scents. Examples include hyacinth, tuberose, lilies, and honeysuckle. It is also manufactured synthetically.

infusion — the process of heating raw materials in a solvent solution to produce an attar.

ionone — an essential compound of violet perfumes and a valued, synthesized product used by the perfumer. Also used in small amounts in floral, woody, and herbaceous scents.

kyphi — the Eygptians' sacred perfume, burned as incense in their temples and homes. An incense paste with a wine and raisin base with aromatic herbs and resins.

leather notes — scents with a smoky aroma characteristic of the ingredients used in the tanning process of leathers. Oil of birch tar and aroma chemicals are used to create leather notes.

light — of a fragrance where the fresh note is predominant. A light fragrance usually is formulated as an eau fraîche.

limbic system — the area in the right side of the brain which receives and interprets fragrance messages. Olfactory nerves, the most primitive brain structure located deep inside the brain, are linked to the limbic system, the seat of our emotions, creativity, sexuality, and memory.

linear fragrance — Instead of the classic perfume structure of top, middle and base notes, linear fragrances produce a strong and instant effect which remains constant. The most common type employs a floral bouquet.

living flower technology — *see* chromatography.

maceration — one of the six methods of obtaining the essence of natural ingredients. Flowers are steeped in vats of hot fat forming pomades which are then washed in alcohol to purify the scented mixture from which an extrait of flower oil is obtained. This process is very similar to enfleurage.

microencapsulation — a technique devised by 3M in 1970 incorporating liquid fragrance oil into a solid, thin-walled capsule. The oil is released when the surface is scratched with a fingernail. This is referred to as "scratch and sniff" and used on fragrance samplers. A dry perfume form is also available.

middle notes — the dominant or heart tones that determine the perfume's family — floral, green, spicy, oriental, chypre, etc. After the top notes fade, about ten minutes after application, the middle notes appear.

milk bath — a fragrant foam, liquid or powdered, containing milk or a milk derivative which provides emollients and moisturizers for the skin when added to the bath.

mossy — describing a scent category with the aromas of a walk through the forest.

mouillette — *see* blotter strip.

mousseline — an Indian perfume based on vetiver. The name is derived from the word muslin, as the fragrance was once used to scent cloth before exportation.

Mysore — a state in southern India where the most valuble sandalwood trees grow.

night bloomer — the growth habit of certain tropical flowers such as honeysuckle, jasmine, and evening primrose, where blooming in daytime heat would cause too much water evaporation for the flower to survive. Night bloomers are very fragrant and light in color.

oceanic — describing a fragrance group evoking the scents of fresh air and ocean breezes.

oriental blend — a composition of exotic, sophisticated scents redolent of sandalwood, vanilla, and musk with warm, powdery notes.

oxidation — the chemical change or alteration of a fragrance and/or its color due to excessive exposure to the air.

ozone — *see* oceanic.

palette — the complete range of raw materials from which the perfumer selects those needed for a particular creation.

perfume — the longest lasting and most concentrated of form of fragrance.

perfumer — often referred to as the "nose" whose imagination and extraordinary sense of smell enable him or her to create harmonious blends.

pheromone — chemicals secreted by animals and insects, influencing behavior of their own or a different species.

pomade — a combination of purified fats and flower oils resulting from enfleurage or maceration.

pomander — an old English term for a perforated ball or box containing fragrant materials. In modern usage, a citrus fruit with cloves rolled in a mix of ground spices and orrisroot powder to preserve it as it dries.

potpourri — a mixture of dry or moist botanicals.

powdery — describing a characteristic trait of perfumes containing heliotropin, vanillin, iris, and tonka beans.

profumego — an ornamental ball used in Italy during the Renaissance and filled with an incense paste. It was hung from a chain or rolled along the floor to perfume a room.

resinoid — any of several extracts of gums, balsams, resins, and roots containing resinous materials. Resinoids are generally used as fixatives in perfume compositions.

resin — any of several gums derived from trees, in particular pine and other evergreens. Commonly used as fixatives.

shower gel — an easy-to-use soap substitute, also good for shaving.

single floral — a fragrance with the scent of a single flower.

smell fingerprint — the individual characteristics of a fragrance creation as it develops on the skin.

soap — the first commercially manufactured soap was in Britain in 1641. Quality perfumed soaps are French-milled for long-lasting hardness.

solvent — a fluid used to extract essential oils from flowers, fruits, resins, herbs, and other natural perfumery materials.

spicy notes — obtained from cinnamon, clove, nutmeg, ginger, cardamom, allspice, lavender, and mace.

sweet — used to describe a fragrance with richness and a vanilla or sugary scent.

synergism — the ability of certain perfumery ingredients to work together to produce an effect greater than the ingredients could achieve independently.

tenacity — the ability of a perfume to last, or a fragrance note to prevail, retaining its characteristic odor.

theme — the dominant accord formulated by the perfumer to give his creation character.

tincture — a prepared perfumery or extract material from alcoholic extracts of raw materials; the solvent is left in the extract as a diluent.

toilet water — a fragrance product less concentrated than eau de parfum; a lighter and more subtle form of fragrance.

top note — the first scent impression of a fragrance, lasting six to ten seconds. Designed to be volatile, often contains citrus notes.

vinaigrette — a small box, usually made of silver, with a pierced inner lid containing a sponge soaked in aromatic vinegar. Popular in Europe through the nineteenth century to counter unpleasant odors in the air and to clear the head.

volatile — having the property of being freely diffused in the atmosphere and easily vaporized at a low temperature. The most volatile notes in the structure of a fragrance are the top notes.

wheat germ oil — an oil with the skin-nourishing properties of vitamin E, along with lecithin and vitamins A and D. Especially good for mature skin and stretch marks. Also used as an anti-bacterial agent in cosmetic preparations.

woodsy-mossy — a forest and fern accord of aromatic woods such as cedar, rosewood, sandalwood and earthy notes of vetiver, oakmoss, patchouli, and fern. Prevalent in men's fragrances and used in women's scents as well.

woody — having the essence of freshly cut wood; cedar, sandalwood, and vetiver provide these notes.

INDEX

A

Absolutes, 17, 157
Accord, 20, 157
Aftershaves, 67
Alcohol base, 3–4, 65, 74, 80
Aldehydes, 12, 98, 157. *See also*
    Modern family
Allspice, 23
Amber, 8, 23, 72. *See also* Oriental
    family
American Star of the Year, 8
Angelica, 24
Animalic, 2, 157
Anise, 24
Apple, 24
Apple slices, preserving, 119
Apricot, 24
Apricot kernel oil, 24
Arden, Elizabeth, 142
Armani, Giorgio, 142
Aroma chemicals, 16–17, 157
Aromacology, 157
Arpège (Lanvin), 4
Ashley, Laura, 142
Attar, 157
Austin, David, 144, 150–51
Azalea, 25

B

Baldwin, King of Constantinople,
    123
Balmain, Pierre, 8
Balms, 67
Balsam of Peru, 25
Base notes, 18–19, 21, 157
Basil, 25
Bath salts, 111
Baudruchage, 157
Bayberry, 25
Bay leaf oil, 25

Beaux, Ernest, 4
Beeswax, 157
Bellanca, Antonia, 142
Benzoin, 26
Bergamot, 26, 72
Bienaimé, 7
Bitter
    almond oil, 26
    orange oil, 26
Black
    currant bud, 26
    pepper, 26–27
Blotter strip, 64, 157
Bois de rose, 27
Borghese, Pauline, 5
Bottles, glass, 6, 69–70, 130
Boucheron, 143
Bouquet, 157
Bousquet, Jean, 143
Bulgari, 143

C

Cacherel, 143
Candlemaker's Companion, The, 128
Cardamom, 27
Carmelite water, 82, 157
Carnation, 27, 72
Caron, 143
Cartier, Jacques, 143
Carven, 143
Cassie, 27
Cassolettes, 125, 158
Castoreum, 27
Catherine de Médici, 3
Cavitch, Susan, 128
Cedarwood oil, 28
Cellier, Germaine, 8
Cellulose, as a base, 118
Chanel, Gabrielle (Coco), 4–5
Chanel No. 5, 4–5, 12–13, 61

Chopard, 144
Chromatography, 21–22, 158
Chypre (Coty), 5
Chypre family
  background, 13, 15
  definition, 158
  fragrance profiles, 55–56
  perfumes, men, 141
  perfumes, women, 138–39
  recipes for, 99–100
Cinnamon, 28
Citronella, 28
Citrus family
  background, 12, 14
  definition, 158
  fragrance profiles, 52–53
  perfumes, men, 140
  recipes for, 96–98
Civet, 28
Claiborne, Liz, 144
Clary sage, 28
Clove bud oil, 29
Coconut oil, 29, 157
Cologne. See also Recipes
  eau de Cologne, 3–4, 66, 81, 158
  shopping for, 64–66
  wearing, how to, 62
Cologne (Germany), 3, 66
Concretes, 17, 158
Containers, 69–71, 130–31. See also
  Packaging
Coriander, 29
Costus, 29
Coty, François, 5, 6, 13
Crabtree & Evelyn, 144
Crafting kits, 75
Cream perfumes, 113–14
Cyclamen, 29

D

Dali, Salvador, 6, 148
Daltroff, Ernest, 143
Damask water, 158
Decorating. See Packaging
Découpage, how to, 131

De La Renta, Oscar, 144
Desprez, Jean, 147
Diffusion, 158
Dior, Christian, 144
Distillation, 16–17
Distilled water, 65, 74, 158
Dramming, 158
Dry
  note, 72, 158
  perfume, 158
Drydown, 18, 21, 158
Dusting powder, 62, 112

E

Earthy note, 72, 158
Eau de Cologne, 3–4, 66, 81, 158
Eau de parfum, 62–66, 74–75, 159
Eau de toilette, 66, 74–75, 159
Eau fraîche, 66, 159. See also Sweet
  Waters
Eau Neuve (Lubin), 5
Elizabeth, Queen of Hungary, 3, 80
Ellis, Perry, 144
Enfleurage, 17, 159
Erox Corporation, 144–45
Essence, 18–21. See also Notes
Essential oils
  for composing perfume, 16–18
  definition, 159
  and fragrance oils, 74, 75–76
  history of, 2
  quality of, 73
  and scent varieties, 66
Eugenol, 29
Evaporation rate, 18, 21, 65
Expression, 17, 159
Extraction, 17, 22, 159
Extrait, 159. See also Perfume

F

Families, fragrance, 10–15, 136–41
Farina, Jean Maria, 3–4
Femme (Rochas), 5, 6
Filtering, 18
Fixatives, 18–19, 159

Flacons (bottles), 6, 159
Floral family
  background, 10, 11
  definition, 159
  fragrance profiles, 54
  perfumes, women, 136–37
  recipes for, 83–86
Florida water, 4, 79
Floriental family
  background, 12
  fragrance profiles, 58–60
  perfumes, women, 138
Flowers
  decorating with, 132–35
  drying, 149
  in fragrance creation, 71
  living flower technology, 21–22
  and scents, 21–22, 149–52
  sources for, 152
Fougère family
  background, 14–15
  definition, 159
  perfumes, men, 140–41
Fragrance. *See also* Cologne; Perfume; Recipes
  burning, 2–4, 114–16
  crafting kits, 75
  creating, how to, 67–75
  definition, 159
  and essential oils, 2, 16–18, 66, 73,
    159
  families, 10–15, 136–41
  ingredients of, 23–46, 67, 71
  longevity of, 47–48, 65–67
  for men, 13–15, 53–61, 66–67,
    140–41
  oils, 74–76, 159
  packaging, 129–35
  for teenagers, 53–57, 61
  wardrobe, 47–64, 159
  for women, 10–13, 53–61, 66,
    136–39
Fragrance Foundation FIFI award, 8
France, 3, 4
Frangipani, 30, 72
Frankincense, 30, 72
Freesia, 30
Fruity family
  background, 11
  definition, 160
  fragrance profiles, 57–58, 61
  perfumes, women, 137–38
  recipes for, 87

G
Galbanum, 30
Gardenias, 30, 151
Geraniums, 31, 133–34
Ginger, 31
Gingham 'n' Spice, Ltd., 9, 75
Givenchy, Hubert de, 145
Gloves, perfumed, 3, 30
Glycerin, 31, 71, 160
Gourmand, 160
Goutal, Annick, 145
Grapefruit, 31
Grasse (France), 3, 160
Green family
  background, 11
  definition, 160
  fragrance profiles, 61
  perfumes, women, 139
  recipes for, 88–89
Guerlain, Jacques, 7–8
Guerlain, Pierre-François, 7
Gum, 31

H
Halston, 145
Hand lotion, 112
Hayfield notes, 160
Haymen, Gale and Fred, 145
Headspace analysis, 21–22, 160
Heart notes, 19–20, 161
Heliotrope, 32, 72
Herbaceous, 160
Hesperidium (citrus), 4, 160
Honey, 32
Honeysuckle, 32
Honey water, 160

Houbigant, Jean-François, 7
Hungary water, 3, 80
Hyacinth, 32

I

Incense, 2–4, 114–16, 160
Indole, 160
Infusion, 160
Ingredients, 23–46, 67, 71. *See also*
   specific ingredients
Insects, 116, 126
International Flavor and Fragrance
   (IFF), 21, 22
Ionone, 160

J

Jasmine, 32–33
Jicky (Guerlain), 7
Jojoba, 33, 75
Jonquil, 33
Joss sticks, 116
Joy (Patou), 6
Juniper, 33

K

Kenzo, 145

L

Labdanum, 8, 33–34
Lagerfeld, Karl, 145–46
L'Air du Temps (Ricci), 6, 7
Lalique, René, 6, 7
Lancaster Group, 144
Lancôme, 146
Lanvin, Jeanne, 4, 13, 14
L'Aphrodite de Cnide (Dali), 6
Lauder, Estée, 8
Lavandin, 34
Lavender, 34, 151
Lavender family, 14, 140
Leather family
  background, 14
  definition, 160
  perfumes, men, 141
Lemongrass, 34

Lemon oil, 34
Ley, Magaretha, 146
Light, 66, 160–61
Lilacs, 34–35, 151
Lily, 35
Lily of the valley, 35
Limbic system, 161
Lime oil, 35
Linaloe oil, 27
Linear fragrance, 161
Living flower technology, 21–22
L'Origan (Coty), 5
Louis XIV, King of France, 3
Lubin, Jean-François, 5

M

Mace, 35
Maceration, 161
Magnolia, 36
Mandarin, 36
Mane, V., 144
Marigold, 36
Maturing, 18
Melon, 36
Men and fragrance
  background, 13–15
  fragrance profiles, 53–61
  fragrance varieties, 66–67
  perfumes, list of, 140–41
  recipes for, 101–4
Metal, avoidance of, 69, 71
Microencapsulation, 161
Middle notes, 19, 20, 161
Miel note, 32
Miglin, Marilyn, 146
Mignonette, 36
Milk bath, 161
Miller, Nicole, 146–47
Millot, 147
Mimosa, 36–37
Miyake, Issey, 147
Modern family. *See also* Aldehydes
  background, 12–13
  fragrance profiles, 59–60
  perfumes, women, 139

Mod Podge, 131
Mookherjee, Braja, 21, 22
Mossy, 161
Mouillette (blotter strip), 64, 157
Mousseline, 161
Mugler, Thierry, 147
Muguet (lily of the valley), 35
Multifloral fragrance, 7
Musical scales and perfume, 18
Musk, 37
Myrrh, 37
Mysore (India), 42, 161

N

Narcissus, 37
Natural oils, 16–18, 73–74
Natural Soap Book, The, 128
Neroli oil, 37, 72
Night bloomers, 161
Night-scented stock, 37
Nose (perfumer), 19, 162
Notes
  base, 21, 157
  and essence, 18–19
  middle, 20, 161
  top, 19–20, 163
Nutmeg, 38

O

Oakmoss, 38, 72
Oceanic family
  background, 13
  complexity of, 101
  definition, 161
  fragrance profiles, 52–53, 61
  perfumes, women, 139
Opoponax, 38
Oppenheimer, Betty, 128
Orange blossom, 38
Orangeflower water, 38, 78
Oriental family
  background, 12
  definition, 161
  fragrance profiles, 60
  perfumes, men, 141

perfumes, women, 138
  recipes for, 92–96
Orris, 38–39
Oscar, 144
Osmanthus, 39
Oxidation, 161
Ozone. *See* Oceanic family

P

Packaging
  bottles, 130
  boxes, 129–30
  flowerpots, 131
  with geraniums, how to, 133–34
  with leaves, how to, 134–35
  with roses, how to, 132–33
Palette, 162
Palma rose oil, 39
Pamplemousse (grapefruit), 31
Pansies, 152
Paraffin, 70
Patchouli, 39, 72
Patou, Jean, 6
Peach, 39
Pear, 39
Penhaligon, William Henry, 147
Pennyroyal, 40
Peppermint, 40
Perfume. *See also* Recipes
  blotter strip for, 64, 157
  classification of, 18
  cologne, compared to, 65–66
  composing, 18–20
  cream, 113–14
  definition, 162
  by fragrance family, 136–41
  and gloves, 3, 30
  history of, 2–8
  single floral, 11, 54, 136, 162
  solid, 113–14
  strength of, 74–75
Perfume King (*Le Roi Parfum*), 3
Perfumer (Nose), 19, 162
Perfumers and their perfumes,
  142–48

Personality and scents, 49–51
Petitgrain, 40
Petitjean, Armand, 146
Pheromones, 144–45, 162
Photosensitivity, 72
Piésse, Septimus, 18
Pineapple, 40
Pine needle oil, 40
Plaid's Decorator Color Blocks, 129
Pleasures (Lauder), 8
Plum, 41
Pomade, 17, 162
Pomanders
  definition, 162
  history of, 123–24
  recipes for, 124
Potpourri
  definition, 162
  history of, 116–17
  recipes for, 117–20
Poucher, W. A., 18
Powdery, 162
Pre-shaves, 67
Profumego, 162
Pulse points, 62, *63*
Punks (joss sticks), 116

Q

Quelques Fleurs (Houbigant), 7

R

Raspberry, 41
Recipes
  Apple Dumpling, 106
  April Showers, 89
  Autumn Leaves, 92
  Basic Spice Mix, 114
  bath salts, 111
  Bay Rum Aftershave, 101
  Baywood, 102
  Bergamot Cologne, 110
  Blushing Rose, 105
  Breath of Spring, 88
  Calming Flower Bath Oil, 112
  Carmelite Water, 82, 157

Citrus Grove, 96
Colonial Rose Potpourri, 117
Cottage Rose Potpourri, 118
Country Kitchen Spice Potpourri,
  117
cream perfumes, 113–14
Crème de Vanille Cologne, 93
Cypress Isle, 99
Deep in the Forest Potpourri,
  120
Delight, 91
dusting powder, 112
Earth Flower, 100
Eau de Cologne, 81
Emerald Herbs, 89
Fireside, 104
Florida Water, 79
Flower Water, 83
Forest, 104
French Sorbet, 109
French Vanilla and Tea Rose
  Perfume, 92
Fruit 'N' Spice, 87
Geranium Toilet Water, 109
Harbor Lights, 103
Herbal Aftershave, 101
Honeybee Sweet Water, 105
Hungary Water, 80
Island Spice Eau de Toilette, 91
Ivy Rose, 95
Key Lime Cologne, 102
Lavender Water, 82
Lemon Verbena Sachet, 121
Linen Cupboard Freshener, 126
Lovenotes, 113
Love's Promise, 85
Melody, 98
Memories, 86
Moonshadow, 100
Mossy Glen, 99
Moth and Insect Repellent, 126
Mulling Spices, 120
Mystery, 94
Nectar, 97
Orangeflower Water, 78

Orchard Fruits, 113
Orient Express, 113
Orris Root Tincture, 78
Paradise, 107
Pearwood, 87
Prom Night, 106
Provence, 103
Rock Garden, 100
Romantic Moments, 113
Rose Cologne, 83
Rose Geranium Sachet, 122
Rose Jar, 85
Rosewater, 77
Rosewater Splash, 76
Scented Furniture Polish, 127
Scented Ink, 127
"Scent Your Own" Sachet Powder, 122
Secrets, 90
Serenity, 108
Silk Shantung, 86
Silky Hand Lotion, 112
solid perfumes, 113–14
Southern Belle, 84
Spice Bath for Pomanders, 124
Spiced Apple Cider Potpourri, 119
Spiced Rosewater, 90
Spice Island, 96
Stillroom Spicy Sachet, 123
Summertime, 98
Sunny Citrus, 114
Sunny Citrus Cologne, 108
Sweet Mystery Incense, 116
Sweet Nothings, 107
Tincture of Benzoin, 78
Tussie Mussie, 93
Valley Green, 113
Verbena Splash, 97
Victorian Rose Burning Perfume, 115
Violet Perfume, 88
Violet Water, 81
Wedding Bliss, 94
Woodlands, 114

Wood Rose, 95
Woodrose Perfume, 84
Woods 'N' Spice Incense, 115
Renaissance, 2
Resins
  definition, 162
  in fragrance, 16, 19, 41
  history of, 2
Ricci, Nina, 6, 7
Rondeletia, 41
Rose bulgare, 41
Rose de mai, 42
Rosemary, 42, 72
Roses, 132–33, 149–50
Rosewater, 42
Rosewood oil, 27
Roudnitska, Edmond, 5, 6, 144
Royal Coat, 131

S

Sachets, 121–23
St. Laurent, Yves, 147
Sandalwood, 42–43, 72
Scents
  for babies, 16
  flowers, 21–22, 149–52
  longevity of, 47–48, 65–67
  men, varieties for, 66–67
  and personality, 49–51
  power of, 9
  shared, 15
  spraying of, 62
  women, varieties for, 66
Schiaparelli, Elsa, 148
Shalimar (Guerlain), 7–8
Shelf life of fragrance, 64
Shower gel, 162
Siberian fir, 43
Single floral perfumes, 11, 54, 136, 162
Skin
  and contaminants, 62
  longevity of scent, 47–48, 65–67
  photosensitivity, 72
  sensitivity testing, 71

Smell and Taste Treatment and
  Research Foundation, 13
Smell fingerprint, 162
Soap, 62, 128, 162
Solid perfumes, 113–14
Solid-Phase Micro Extraction, 22
Solvent extraction, 17, 162
Spicy family
  background, 2, 11, 14
  definition, 162
  fragrance profiles, 55, 56
  perfumes, men, 140
  perfumes, women, 139
  recipes for, 90–92
Star anise, 43
Stephanotis, 43
Storage of ingredients, 67, 71
Styrax, 43
Sung, Alfred, 148
Sun King (Le Roi Soleil), 3
Sweet
  almond oil, 43
  bags, 121–23
  definition, 162
  orange, 44
  peas, 44, 151
Sweet waters, 17, 74–75. See also
  Recipes
Synergism, 162
Synthetic oils, 16–18, 73–74

T

Talcs, 67
Tangerine, 44
Teenagers and fragrance, 53–57, 61,
  105–8
Tenacity, 162
Tenax trap, 22
Theme, 162
Thyme, 44
Tiffany, 148
Tincture, 163
Toilet water, 15, 62, 64, 163
Tonka bean, 44
Top notes, 18–20, 163

Tuberose, 45, 72
Turkey red oil, 45

U

Unisex fragrances, 15, 108–10, 141

V

Van Cleef & Arpels, 148
Vanilla, 45, 72
Vanillin, 45
Ventilation, 67
Vent Vert (Balmain), 8
Verbena, 45
Vetiver, 45–46, 72
Victoria, Queen of England, 15
Vinaigrettes, 125, 163
Violets, 46, 151
Vodka, use of, 74
Volatile, 163

W

Wardrobe, fragrance, 47–64, 159
Water, distilled, 65, 74, 158
Water lily, 46
Wheat germ oil, 46, 163
Women and fragrance. See also
  Recipes
  background, 10–13
  fragrance profiles, 53–61
  fragrance varieties, 66
  perfumes, list of, 135–39
Woodsy-mossy, 163
Woody family
  background, 15
  definition, 163
  perfumes, men, 140

Y

Ylang-ylang, 46
Youth Dew (Lauder), 8

OTHER STOREY TITLES YOU WILL ENJOY

The Aromatherapy Companion, by Victoria H. Edwards.
The most comprehensive aromatherapy guide, filled with profiles
of essential oils and recipes for beauty, health, and well-being.
288 pages. Paper. ISBN 978-1-58017-150-2.

The Essential Oils Book: Creating Personal Blends for Mind & Body,
by Colleen K. Dodt.
A rich resource on the many uses of aromatherapy and its applications in
everyday life.
160 pages. Paper. ISBN 978-0-88266-913-7.

The Herbal Home Remedy Book, by Joyce A. Wardwell.
A wealth of herbal healing wisdom, with advice on how to collect and store
herbs, make remedies, and stock a home herbal medicine chest.
176 pages. Paper. ISBN 978-1-58017-016-1.

**The Herbal Home Spa: Naturally Refreshing Wraps, Rubs, Lotions,
Masks, Oils, and Scrubs,** by Greta Breedlove.
A collection of easy-to-create personal care products that rival potions
found at exclusive spas and specialty shops.
208 pages. Paper. ISBN 978-1-58017-005-5.

The Natural Soap Book: Making Herbal and Vegetable-Based Soaps,
by Susan Miller Cavitch.
Basic recipes for soaps made without chemical additives and synthetic
ingredients, as well as ideas on scenting, coloring, cutting, trimming,
and wrapping soaps.
192 pages. Paper. ISBN 978-0-88266-888-8.

Organic Body Care Recipes, by Stephanie Tourles.
Homemade, herbal formulas for glowing skin, hair, and nails,
plus a vibrant self.
384 pages. Paper. 978-1-58017-676-7.

The Soapmaker's Companion, by Susan Miller Cavitch.
A resource for beginner and advanced soapmakers alike, from
mastering basic skills to creating soaps with a personal touch.
288 pages. Paper. ISBN 978-0-88266-965-6.

These and other books from Storey Publishing are available
wherever quality books are sold or by calling 1-800-441-5700.
Visit us at *www.storey.com*.